Diets don't work...
but Jesus does!

Inner-healing, permanent weight loss and spiritual breakthrough based on the living Word of God.

Shannon Tanner
Founder,
Body Temple Wellness Workshops

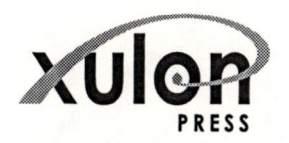

xulon
PRESS

Copyright © 2007 by Shannon Tanner

Diets don't work...but Jesus does!
by Shannon Tanner

Printed in the United States of America

ISBN-13: 978-1-60034-965-2
IBSN-10: 1-60034-965-X

All rights reserved solely by the author. The author guarantees all contents are original and do not infringe upon the legal rights of any other person or work. No part of this book may be reproduced in any form without the permission of the author. The views expressed in this book are not necessarily those of the publisher.

Unless otherwise noted, Scripture quotations are taken from the Holy Bible New King James Version. Copyright © 1982 by Thomas Nelson, Inc.

www.xulonpress.com

*This book is dedicated to my husband, Bryan Tanner.
A servant, leader, confidant and tireless supporter of all I do.
I love you and I am dedicated to building a Kingdom empire
with you, both now and forever.*

TABLE OF CONTENTS

Acknowledgements ix

Preface - The *overweight* Weight Loss Specialist xi

Introduction - *Diets don't work… but Jesus does* xiii

Chapter One - Recognition 23

Chapter Two - Recognize True Hunger 31

Chapter Three - Overcoming Overeating 41

Chapter Four - Your Body is a Temple 49

Chapter Five - Wise Eating 55

Chapter Six - How Faith Changes Shape 69

Chapter Seven - Seeking God's Hand and Not My Own 83

Chapter Eight - Living in the Moment 89

Chapter Nine – Self-Love for Weight Loss Success 97

Chapter Ten - How Faith Wins at Weight Loss 107

Chapter Eleven - Worship Over Weight 117

Chapter Twelve - Slim and Serene by Submission 125

Acknowledgements

I would like to thank the courageous women of Body Temple Wellness. Your testimonies, strength, support and humility continue to inspire me. To Pastor Monique Robinson for being a light on my path; I bless God for your insight, leadership and love. This book would not be without you. To Bishop Ulmer, First Lady Togetta Ulmer and the entire family of Faithful Central Bible Church for providing me with a platform to share my gifts with the Body of Christ. Your teachings and generosity have blessed me beyond measure! To Pastors Brian and Tara Lewis, your passionate pursuit of God has been the driving force behind my own quest for all God has for me! To my father, L.J. Martin, for the gift of words, the power of belief and creative ingenuity. To my mother, Orngiel Martin, for the gift of passion, fire and boldness in Christ! To my Pastor Frank Wilson for teaching me to never limit the power of God in my life and for challenging me to walk in renewed purpose and excellence. To the entire New Dawn Christian Village family, thank you for loving me and my family the way that you do. To my three wonderful boys: Joshua, Josiah and Joseph, mommy is blessed by your unconditional affection, love and faith. To my princess, Jade, and Sir Tyler, your auntie loves you both with all of her heart. You two have given me the gift of your adoration and wisdom. To my editor, Daphne McVay, thank you for your dedication, honesty, love and support, you were my spiritual mid-wife and your diligence helped to birth this great vision. Finally, to sister Bunny Wilson for teaching me the gift of surrender and for being my most powerful example of perfect strength and dependence on God. Your Godly beauty, influence and discernment so wonderfully amaze me.

PREFACE

The *Overweight* Weight Loss Specialist

Before you begin reading the revolutionary and life-changing principles of this book, I need to confess to you that most of the years I spent publicly as a weight loss counselor in the *secular* diet industry, I spent privately in shame as a habitual overeater and food addict.

In my years in the commercial weight loss field, I held many titles including top sales representative, program director, weight loss counselor, lifestyle teacher/coach, center manager and even national television spokesperson for one of the top commercial weight loss centers in the world. Yet secretly, I battled the overwhelming and painful struggle of emotional and disordered eating. It was not until I was introduced to the powerfully healing and transforming Word of God that my body and life were permanently changed!

I look back on how ridiculous the concept of managing weight and food was, and on how for years I lived bound with the fantasy of finding the "quick fix" or the miracle formula when all the while, the truth was inside of me. When I stopped crying out for God to change my body and surrendered my life to Him, I was released from the bondage of human limitation. I began to lose the *inner weights* of shame, guilt, fear and pride that had kept me bound in a cycle of compulsive eating. I made a choice to take my eyes off of myself and fix them on Jesus. It is my prayer that as you read this book, you will allow yourself the freedom to step boldly in your deliverance, freedom and victory. I pray that you would move out of your own way of success and wake up to the truth that the food is not the enemy, we are. We have stood in the way of Godly restoration, success and greatness for far too long. The Lord has a wonderful plan for your health, wealth, purpose and passion. Allow yourself to start a diet of consuming God's love and experience incredible and undeniable results that prove…

Diets don't work…but Jesus does!

INTRODUCTION

Diets don't work... but Jesus does!

*L*ast year, we spent an estimated $46 billion on diet products and self-help books. It is estimated that two-thirds of American dieters regained all the weight that they had lost within a year and up to 99% of dieters gain it all back within five years. The 46 billion dollar diet industry that encompasses everything from e-coaching to shakes and pills to medical weight loss centers, is the only booming and rapidly growing industry in the world where 97-99% of customers fail. And since weight loss centers are not required by government law to provide weight loss outcomes or data supporting their program success rates, it remains one of the only unregulated industries where the actual product is never checked for consumer effectiveness. As a matter of fact, the very livelihood of the weight loss industry is built upon consumer failure. If people were to permanently lose weight, the entire industry would fail! Close to 75% of enrollments at commercial weight loss centers are returning customers! It is no secret that we as Americans, and the entire world for that matter, are becoming more obese each year. For all of our infomercials, weight loss gurus and countless diet methods, we continue to repeat the cycle of weight loss and weight gain, essentially failing year after year. Christians are not an exception to this rule. In many ways, they are leading the number in statistics on obesity and illness. God called us to be a light unto the world and to show wisdom, not to follow in the world's pattern of confusion. When we are dieting, we become familiar with failure.

When we trust God, we soon discover that there is only one thing God cannot do...fail!

When we follow wholeheartedly after the Word of God and the steps of Jesus, we will experience lasting change and freedom. There is no limit to the Word of God and its life-changing power! This book was not written for someone who wants to drop a few pounds by Christmas to see the family or squeeze back into the bikini for summer. This book is for people who want lasting freedom from overeating and poor health. *Diets don't work... but Jesus does* was written for those who want to be totally restored in mind, body and spirit.

Why Diets Don't Work

Diets focus on food management not heart change

Colossians 2:20-23 Therefore, if you died with Christ from the basic principles of the world, why, as though living in the world, do you subject yourselves to regulations "Do not touch, do not taste, do not handle," which all concern things which perish with the using—according to the commandments and doctrines of men? These things indeed have an appearance of wisdom in self-imposed religion, false humility, and neglect of the body, but are of no value against the indulgence of the flesh.

Whether it's good carbs, bad carbs, no carbs, glycemic index, high protein liquid, vegan, Mediterranean diet, Hollywood diet or one of the other thousands of plans or programs, they simply take a different angle and use their own signature marketing to package the only tried and true weight loss method, which is eat less and move more! What we will prove to you in the teachings of *Diets don't work... but Jesus does* is that outside regulations and food management have no power to heal the heart of the overeater. These strict outside regimens appeal to our deep pain as overeaters because they offer us short term relief from the fear of food. When we make food our focus, we continue on the cycle of deprivation, guilt and overeating. When we realize that true change lies within us, not outside of us, we will lay down the heavy burden of looking outside of ourselves for help. We will know that God has everything we need. When God places a desire for change in our hearts, He equips us with the tools, wisdom and self-control to see the vision come to pass.

Diets prove we can not keep the law

Galatians 3:11-13 But that no one is justified by the law in the sight of God is evident, for "the just shall live by faith." Yet the law is not of faith, but "the man who does them shall live by them." Christ has redeemed us from the curse of the law, having become a curse for us for it is written, "Cursed is everyone who hangs on a tree"

When do most people start a diet? On Monday! What do we do over the weekend before we start our diet? We binge! We eat everything we will not have while we are on our next *miracle* weight loss plan. We make vows and pledge our loyalty to the new meal plan. But what happens when we break the law of our new diet? We mentally beat on ourselves. I binge, beat myself up and start all over again. Some people live their entire lives going from a diet to an eating binge to another diet and never get off of this self-defeating cycle. Dieting opens the door for an eating disorder. Diet laws prove to me that I cannot keep the law. I need the supernatural power of the Holy Spirit. Willpower has failed me time and time again and it's time for liberty, freedom and grace, not diet laws!

Diets conform, God transforms

Romans 12:1-2 I beseech you therefore, brethren, by the mercies of God, that you present your bodies a living sacrifice, holy, acceptable to God, which is your reasonable service. And do not be conformed to this world, but be transformed by the renewing of your mind, that you may prove what is the good and acceptable and perfect will of God.

When I diet, I am conforming to this world. I am doing what the world is doing, trying to control myself by outward regulations and food manipulation. God wants to give us new thoughts, not have us follow the limited wisdom of man. When God renews our mind through His Holy Word, we will gain the victory. When we diet, our entire focus is on changing our bodies. God desires to change *us*. Once our hearts are changed through His Word, our bodies will soon follow.

Diets place our trust in the wrong method for victory

2 Corinthians 10:4 For though we walk in the flesh, we do not war according to the flesh. For the weapons of our warfare are not carnal but mighty in God for pulling down strongholds

Dieting ensures our failure and frustration because our trust is in the wrong place for healing and freedom. When we fight the battle of the flesh with the carnal weapon of dieting we are defeated by our own futile efforts. We are in a spiritual battle. Waving a meal planner at the enemy is like fighting a forest fire with a child's water gun. When we learn to employ the spiritual weapons of prayer, fasting, worship, daily faith/action and obedience, all of the power of heaven comes to our aid. We are prepared to stand against the enemy and gain victory over our own body when we walk by the spirit.

Dieting puts my trust in the wrong place

Jeremiah 17: 5-8 Thus says the LORD: Cursed is the man who trusts in man and makes flesh his strength, whose heart departs from the LORD. For he shall be like a shrub in the desert, and shall not see when good comes, but shall inhabit the parched places in the wilderness, in a salt land which is not inhabited. Blessed is the man who trusts in the LORD, and whose hope is the LORD. For he shall be like a tree planted by the waters, which spreads out its roots by the river, and will not fear when heat comes; but its leaf will be green, and will not be anxious in the year of drought, nor will cease from yielding fruit.

When I diet, I mentally coach myself and say, "I'm going to do it this time!" "This is the plan!" We put so much focus on self. But the

Bible says, "Cursed is the man who trusts in man and makes flesh his strength" (Jeremiah 17:5). When I transfer my trust and seek God's help, I am blessed instantly! When I trust God, I recognize that the source of my strength does not lie outside of me in a plan or program. My true strength is within... the presence of God's Holy Spirit operating powerfully through me.

Why Jesus Works!

With Jesus, the yo-yo dieting cycle is broken

John 15:5 "I am the vine, you are the branches. He who abides in me, and I in him, bears much fruit; for without Me you can do nothing.

I can try my agenda or program, but God calls me to acknowledge Him in all of my ways and He will show me success. The reason for my repeated dieting failure is simply that I have been performing and fighting to earn my weight loss success instead of *trusting* to receive God's direction, wisdom and provision that leads to lasting stability and peace. The greatest leaders and visionaries of the Bible <u>never</u> sought success alone, they sought *whole-heartedly* after God, and their success was inevitable!

Jesus empowers us through fellowship not diet isolation

1 John 1:7 But if we walk in the light as He is in the light, we have fellowship with one another, and the blood of Jesus Christ His Son cleanses us from all sin.

The enemy will always attack the sheep that has strayed away from the flock. The principle of fellowship, transparency and confessing our sins to one another is a godly command. We cannot do it on our own, we need one another. In small group fellowship, we are encouraged by the testimonies of victory and are refreshed when we minister and share with others. Fellowship is the will of God. When we gather together in His name, He is in the midst (Matthew 18:20). Even in the secular realm, the most successful, commercial weight loss centers employ the godly principle of group accountability. I encourage you to partner in a small group study as you go through the teachings in this book so that you can celebrate the victory in the lives of other believers as you journey towards your new life and victory.

Jesus gives us lasting freedom, not short term results

John 8:-36 Therefore if the Son makes you free, you shall be free indeed.

This book is for people who want freedom. God gave us dominion over everything in this earth, including our bodies. Food makes a wonderful servant, but a horrible master. We have bowed down to the limited and deceptive comfort of food for too long. Jesus died on the cross that we would experience lasting freedom in our earthly lives. We have the ability to tap into the resurrection power of Calvary and experience true liberty. If your hope has been destroyed by diet failure, God wants to restore you to a place of promise and blessing.

Jesus offers unconditional love and forgiveness, not diet guilt and deprivation

Colossians 2:13-17 And you, being dead in your trespasses and the uncircumcision of your flesh, He has made alive together with Him, having forgiven you all trespasses, having wiped out the handwriting of requirements that was against us, which was contrary to us. And He has taken it out of the way, having nailed it to the cross. Having disarmed principalities and powers, He made a public spectacle of them, triumphing over them in it. So let no one judge you in food or in drink, or regarding a festival or a new moon or Sabbaths, which are a shadow of things to come, but the substance is of Christ.

Jesus died to set us free from the bondage of legalism. Diet guilt does not motivate us to change; it does the opposite. As emotional eaters, it only furthers the cycle of food abuse. The enemy hides in legalism and religion. The guilt cycle of *religious* Christians and dieters only proves to be self-defeating. God is not examining the size of our bodies; He is looking at the size of our hearts. Can we accept the forgiveness and grace that He has for our lives? I challenge you to step out of the heavy bondage of guilt and shame and receive the unconditional love that will motivate you to a place of true healing.

In Jesus, my weight loss success is promised

Romans 8:37 Yet in all these things we are more than conquerors through Him who loved us.

Studies have shown that people who have more than 75 pounds of weight to lose have less than a 1% chance of losing it and keeping it off. But we serve a God that delights in the impossible. God's Living Word propels us to life-changing daily faith/action. When I realize and accept that I am more than a conqueror and that the battle has already been won, I can move into the realm of manifesting and seeing tangible results in my daily life. My weight loss victory becomes a visible testimony to the greatness of God's healing power in my life.

I trust that God has already prepared your heart for the freedom and victory that lies ahead. He is challenging us all to take Him fully at His Word, to lay down our own destructive weapons of self-sabotage and allow ourselves the privilege, honor and birthright of freedom, confidence and success! Jesus promised us the abundant life in the Bible and that includes our body and health. New life begins when we recognize where the source of our strength lies. The power of surrender is a liberating force in your walk toward weight loss and wellness. When we choose to lay down our heaviness on the inside, the Word of God transforms us and we reflect that change on the outside because *Diets don't work...but Jesus does!*

CHAPTER ONE

Recognition

2 Chronicles 7:14 If My people who are called by My name will humble themselves, and pray and seek My face, and turn from their wicked ways, then I will hear from heaven, and will forgive their sin and heal their land. Now My eyes will be open and My ears attentive to prayer *made* in this place.

It was God's desire that His people know that His house was to be a place of reverence, repentance and honor. The Old Testament temple that Solomon spent seven years of his life constructing was a place of absolute splendor, majesty and beauty. No expense was spared in the constructing of the temple. It is believed by some biblical scholars that re-creating that same temple today would cost in excess of 20 million dollars. Thirty thousand skilled workers were employed by King Solomon and seven years were invested to build a temple that one high priest could go into one time per year to pray for repentance for the sins of God's people. And yet, we have been given a temple (our body) where we have access to God's precious and powerful Holy Spirit every moment of our existence. Is it any wonder that we should have more reverence, honor and respect offered to God in His dwelling place…our bodies?

1 Corinthians 6:19 Or do you not know that your body is the temple of the Holy Spirit *who is* in you, whom you have from God, and you are not your own?

The Word of God clearly reveals to us that our bodies are the temples of the Holy Spirit. The same instructions that Solomon was given in the Old Testament about the temple will be applied in our quest for victory and healing: *one*-humility, *two*-prayer, *three*-turning to God's wisdom instead of our own limited understanding. These steps will bring about life change and lasting weight loss.

When we choose God, our transformation begins

God is waiting on us. It's our move and the transformation starts within our hearts. He's waiting on us to turn away from our own ways and to turn our lives completely over to Him. He's waiting on us to recognize our weakness, to recognize our need for a Sovereign and Almighty God to come in and be our strength in the struggle. Recognition of our need for God does not mean we stop moving forward in daily action, it simply means as we move and step out by faith we recognize the source of our power.

It's time to transfer our trust

If you want to end your struggle with overeating and poor health then it is time to stop putting your trust in the systems of this world that have only led you to failure and frustration. True change happens when we make a decision to allow the fullness of God's power to operate in our lives. We, as believers *box God in*, and limit Him to what *we can see* ourselves achieving. When we admit our weakness, we have access to His perfect strength.

2 Corinthians 12:9 And He said to me, "My grace is sufficient for you, for My strength is made perfect in weakness." Therefore most gladly I will rather boast in my infirmities, that the power of Christ may rest upon me.

I want God's grace and so I choose to humble myself

James 4:6 But He gives more grace. Therefore He says: *"God resists the proud, But gives grace to the humble."*

It's a wonderfully bittersweet time when you come to the place in your life where you are down on your knees, broken in all the right places, saying to a Sovereign, Holy and all-knowing Lord, "God, I cannot do this anymore, I NEED you!" For some of us, getting to that place of humility and repentance may take a lifetime. For others, it only takes a moment to recognize the foolishness of the cycle that we've been on, the insanity that we've subjected ourselves to when we keep doing the same thing over and over and over again and expecting a different result.

Matthew 23:12 And whoever exalts himself will be humbled, and he who humbles himself will be exalted.

I remember this exact crossroads in my own life. I had been an expert in the weight loss field for many years, but still could not get my own eating habits under control. I felt out of control, consumed with thoughts of food, dieting and weight loss. And although I could draft nutrition plans, tell you the fat grams and carbohydrate count of most foods and recite how many calories were burned during any given activity, I was hopeless on the inside. With all of my knowledge, I was still failing and still gaining weight year after year.

When I fell to my knees and admitted that I couldn't hold it all together, I wept before God and asked so desperately and earnestly for His help. A new and profound peace came over me. I knew from that moment forward that my life would be different. I felt a heavy burden was lifted from me that day and I knew God was going to transform my entire life!

God delights in doing the impossible

Luke 1:37 For with God nothing will be impossible.

We serve a God who by His words formed all of creation. There is no limit to His power to transform our lives. He is waiting on us to acknowledge our need and receive His supernatural provision and grace. Overcoming overeating is a lifetime of acknowledging our desire to please God more than ourselves. It is a lifetime of recognizing our need for His wisdom and direction. It is a lifetime of surrendering to His perfect will and not our own.

Choosing God, is Choosing freedom

When we jump on the latest weight loss bandwagon of the world, seek the latest fad diet, quick fix or temporary cure, we may experience hope for a moment, but we most often end up disillusioned and disappointed. When we make it our belief that the next revolutionary weight loss program, that latest infomercial, that next food restrictive food regimen will bring our deliverance, we can miss the quiet, loving voice of a Holy God. God is our deliverance. God is our healing balm and our freedom from the shame and pain of obesity. We just need to turn to Him. When we seek God in this and every struggle that we face, we receive a peace that passes all understanding as His gift to us.

Philippians 4:6-7 Be anxious for nothing, but in everything by prayer and supplication, with thanksgiving, let your requests be made known to God; and the peace of God, which surpasses all understanding, will guard your hearts and minds through Christ Jesus.

God will give us the joy and strength needed for this journey when we turn our hearts fully to Him. He will exalt us to a place of healthy well-being when we fix our eyes on His Word. He will exalt us to that place of energy, power, endurance and longevity promised in the Bible. He will deliver us from our *own works* and set our feet on a new ground. Are you ready to break the cycle? Are you ready for God's blessings? Then let us take the first step and recognize how much we need Him.

Health is the cornerstone of prosperity

Health is one of the most abundant blessings that we can have. Whether it's running after your kids at the park and not getting tired, walking up a flight of stairs without being out of breath or not having to be forced to buy everything that you wear from one side of the store, it is a blessing to have choice and freedom. Prosperity is found in a mastering your body and not a being a servant to it. Having God's blessing in our health is not having the excess flesh that we've put on, but it's having the excess and abundance of God's spirit and His glory. When people see our reflection, they won't see *our* provision. They will not see our gluttony and fear. Instead, when they see us, they will witness *God's glory* moving in and through our lives because there's something sweet and beautiful about surrender.

Surrender starts the process of healing and breakthrough

It's a decision that we make and all of Heaven will shift in our favor to assist us when we recognize our need for God. Recognition is one of the most powerful principles in life. The man of your dreams can be right in your midst, but if you fail to recognize him then you continue to be alone. Likewise, the ultimate plan for victory can be within reach, but if we fail to recognize it, then we continue on a yo-yo cycle up and down, never attaining the stabilizing power of Christ. The day my life changed as a sinner was the day I recognized my need for Christ. Although eternal change occurred within that moment that I asked Jesus Christ to be my personal Lord and Savior, the Bible says we need to recognize Him *daily*.

Philippians 2:12 Therefore, my beloved, as you have always obeyed, not as in my presence only, but now much more in my absence, work out your own salvation with fear and trembling

Our deep need for God

We don't need God just one time or to bail us out of emergencies every once in awhile. We need Him minute-by-minute, day-by-day.

In order to put an end to this struggle with overeating and obesity, we need Him even more. We need to hear His voice even more. We need His comfort and wisdom daily. Recognition of my need for God's power and obedience to the wisdom provided in His Word is what brought about my 73 pound weight loss victory. Continuing daily to surrender my pain and struggle to a loving Heavenly Father is what has kept the weight off for over ten years!

Proverbs 28:26 He who trusts in his own heart is a fool, but whoever walks wisely will be delivered.

Throughout this book, I'm going to teach you how to walk wisely, listen to God's voice, pay attention to and care for the wonderful body that He has given you. You'll learn how to get your body stronger, healthier and leaner, all without dieting, but by simply following the wisdom that is so carefully and perfectly laid out in God's Word.

James 1:5 If any of you lacks wisdom, let him ask of God, who gives to all liberally and without reproach, and it will be given to him.

I believe that if you're reading this book that you are already preparing your heart and mind for what God has in store. I believe, by faith, that you are ready to trust God for your healing and restoration. You can choose to begin a new life today, a life of wellness, strength and vibrant energy. I used to cry out to God, "If you would only change my body then my life would be different." But God was saying, "If you let me change your life then your body will follow."

God alone gets the glory for my weight loss success!

God and God alone receives my praise for bringing me out of my own darkness of obesity, overeating and poor health into His marvelous light of lasting transformation in my mind, body and spirit! God helped me get the victory over my own self sabotage.

Romans 12:1-3 I beseech you therefore, brethren, by the mercies of God, that you present your bodies a living sacrifice, holy, acceptable to God, *which is* your reasonable service. And do not be conformed to this world, but be transformed by the renewing of your mind, that you may prove what *is* that good and acceptable and perfect will of God. For I say, through the grace given to me, to everyone who is among you, not to think *of himself* more highly than he ought to think, but to think soberly, as God has dealt to each one a measure of faith.

God is more than enough

God has provided through His word everything that we need for deliverance. In God's presence we find inner-healing and peace. Through God's daily direction and wisdom we step into a place of lasting results and permanent weight loss. Applying God's natural laws help us move into a new level of wellness. True joy comes when I realize that there is NOTHING God and I cannot handle. God is MORE than enough. Do you recognize your need for Him?

I realize that some of you reading this book may not have a personal relationship with the Lord and Savior Jesus Christ that I write about. If that's you and you're ready to recognize His place in your life and your need for Him on this journey, then I want you to say this prayer with me.

Dear Lord, forgive me, for I am a sinner. I invite You into my heart and I invite You into my life. I believe that You died on the cross and that You rose again. I turn my back on the ways of this world and I turn my back on the sin in which I was living. I ask to begin a new journey with You today. Lord Jesus, please come into my heart and my life and become my Savior. I pray all these things in Your name. Amen.

New Beginnings

For those of you who are on your journey toward daily recognition and surrender, I congratulate you. I'm so excited for you because your life, from this moment on, will never be the same. Look forward with eager expectation to walking in victory. Look forward to walking in deliverance. Look forward to knowing in your heart that *DIETS DON'T WORK...BUT JESUS DOES*!

God has the ultimate success plan for you, your health and your well being. Are you ready to recognize Him?

CHAPTER TWO

Recognize True Hunger

Experts say that food addiction is the hardest addiction to break

It is the one addiction that cannot be cured by going "cold turkey." We have to eat to live. Almost anywhere we go, we're reminded of our struggle. Every corner, every highway and even our social events are all centered on food, our *drug* of choice. The facts prove that close to 97 percent of overweight dieters will remain overweight dieters on a constant swing from loss to gain, gain to loss and the cycle continues. But there's a way to overcome what some people say is impossible.

Where our true battle lies

The only reason we have lost this battle in the past is because we haven't had the right weapons. When we take our eyes off of self, then we'll be free to see Jesus in all of His glory. You're not a failure. You have simply been fighting this battle using the wrong weapons.

2 Corinthians 10:4 For the weapons of our warfare *are* not carnal but mighty in God for pulling down strongholds

Bondage to food and the appetite of the flesh is a stronghold. Fighting a spiritual battle with a carnal (man made) weapon doesn't work. Remember Dracula? I remember in those classic movies, there were only certain things that could kill him, a silver bullet or a stake through the heart.

If you try to kill Dracula in any other way, then your attempts are useless. It is the same way with us. We've been fighting a battle with the wrong weapons because the weapons of our warfare are not *of* this world. They are powerful. They are mighty and bring on lasting victory. The moment we put our trust in Jesus, our victory becomes a reality.

Absolute victory is found in Christ!

This is bigger than a smaller dress size. This is more important than that summer bikini. This is more fabulous than that pair of jeans that you want to fit into again. This is more exciting than the 20 pounds you need to drop before your best friend's wedding or high-school reunion. The goal that we are going after is lasting victory and life-long freedom! Our goal is glorifying God in our temples. When we put our trust in Him, our life vision will become a reality. For absolute victory, we need the proper information. We're embarking on a journey, where we will learn to trust in God's perfect system.

Psalm 139:14 I will praise You, for I am fearfully *and* wonderfully made; Marvelous are Your works, And *that* my soul knows very well.

Hunger vs. Appetite

God placed in us a natural system to regulate hunger, which in turn will regulate and maintain our true and desired weight. On this journey, we will always experience two types of hunger: *true physical hunger* and <u>false hunger</u> or *appetite*. Most overweight people eat from *appetite* and have lost sensitivity to the sensation and regulatory direction of true physical hunger. You will learn in this chapter how to discern and respond to true hunger, which is the first step in natural eating and weight loss.

God's natural weight loss plan

True physical hunger is something that God put in us as a natural function of our bodies to ensure survival. It's how animals survive. They are led and respond to true physical hunger. Have you ever seen an overweight animal *in the wild*? Domesticated animals are overweight because they're fed by people. They, like many of us, have been taught that food is equal to love. Animals in the wild know when they're hungry and when they are full and because of this, their weight is regulated. True physical hunger is a core signal that God designed for our physical nourishment, weight stability, energy regulation and health.

Where does false hunger come from?

False hunger or appetite stems from our habits, compulsive responses to our external environment and oftentimes a basic inability to discern what our spirit and emotions truly need. We can get into a life pattern of confusing feelings, sensations, emotions and the need for safety and comfort with a need to reach for food. Eating from false hunger/appetite not only taxes our bodily organs, but this overeating stresses us and ages us prematurely. From a spiritual viewpoint, eating in bondage from appetite/false hunger can keep us from experiencing dynamic spiritual growth and breakthrough. When we develop a habit of feeding our physical bodies with more priority than feeding our spirit through prayer, fasting, worship, fellowship and biblical meditation, we create lean spirits and bulging bodies.

It's time to create fat spirits and lean bodies

When we start to focus on the root of our hunger, the empty cry of our souls which long for intimacy with a loving, gracious and all-knowing God, we will begin to lose the *inner weights* and the *outer weight* will follow. What prompts our reach for food will be more important on this journey than knowing the carbohydrate and calorie count of what we are eating. The *diet mentality* puts all of the focus on the foods we consume, but God looks at the heart and soul.

1 Samuel 16:7 But the LORD said to Samuel, "Do not look at his appearance or at his physical stature, because I have refused him. For *the LORD does* not *see* as man sees; for man looks at the outward appearance, but the LORD looks at the heart."

Weight loss naturally

We'll be following a simple method for natural eating restoration. We will wait on, and respond only to true physical hunger. Our bodies are in a place of self-healing. If I were to cut myself, my body would heal the wound. Likewise, the overweight body is in a state of *dis-ease*. The excess weight and fat storage taxing the heart, joints and organs is something that the body is willing and eager to correct.

Eat less...lose more

The way that the body will restore health and balance is through *less eating*. No matter how many diet fads or exercise regimens come and go, there is only one way to lose weight and keep it off. You must burn more energy/calories than your body consumes. It's just that simple. Through our Body Temple Wellness workshops, our participants began to lose weight instantly after embracing and practicing the principle of responding only to true hunger. When we rely on the principle of true hunger response and put this new behavior into diligent practice, we will activate our bodies' natural defense system against obesity and the weight will melt away. Listen for, wait on and respond only to true physical hunger and you will eat less. This practice will become a *natural* appetite suppressant and you will begin to shed the pounds.

What is false hunger or appetite?

False hunger usually stems from external situations, habits and surroundings. False hunger is impulsive and driven by external cues such as the purchases you make in the checkout line at the grocery store. "I see it then I *want* it." Appetite is based on bodily senses such as smell and sight. It can also be stimulated by the environment.

Appetite by the clock

It's 9:00 a.m. At 9:00 a.m., everybody always goes down to the food truck. So instantly, I start to feel hungry. That's learned/false hunger. It's 12:00 p.m. and lunch time, or it's 8:00 p.m. and my favorite TV show is on so it's time for me to grab a snack.

Appetite motivated by people

They say that children struggle with peer pressure. Adults succumb to their own form of peer pressure. "Hey, let's go grab a bite to eat," and just to fit in with the crowd, to be accepted, to feel that tiny bit of love that you get from going along with a crowd, you'll sit down and eat, numbing yourself with food, appeasing your flesh. All the while, appetite is sitting at the helm of the controls. What about eating buddies? I used to have an eating buddy. As soon as I saw her, I would get hungry because we always went out together to eat. *People, places, times, foods and moods* can trigger in us what's called a *learned hunger*, but it is false hunger and it leads to weight gain.

Appetite driven by a need for comfort

For many of us, when we were little kids, we didn't have a safe place. We never felt protected, and food became a reliable source of comfort for us. So now, whenever we need to feel safe, connected or loved, we reach for temporary comfort through food. When we experience emotions that we cannot name such as anger, shame or guilt, we run to food because it's familiar. The diet world puts an emphasis on managing and manipulating our food yet what we truly need is healing in our hearts. We need a safe place to validate, move through and experience our emotions. I believe that when we learn with God's help to process, embrace, share and express our feelings and not bury them in food, we will be the most powerful, discerning, expressive and creative people that this world has yet to see.

Psalm 71:21 You shall increase my greatness and comfort me on every side.

Lasting satisfaction

Our true hunger is often for God's fellowship and His presence. When we start to feed ourselves on God's Word instead of food, we will begin to feel fulfillment and satisfaction that most people will never choose to know. But in order to do this, we must take the first natural step to weight loss and healing, which is learning to recognize and respond to true physical hunger.

How do I begin to wait on and respond to true physical hunger?

True hunger is regulated by your *body's need for energy*. A calorie is a unit of energy. True hunger is an unmistakable urge, physical sensation, emptiness and hollow feeling from our stomach that calls loudly for fulfillment.

How does true hunger feel?

True physical hunger is a feeling so strong that it cannot be mistaken. It is the feeling that prompted Esau to give up his birthright in the Bible.

Genesis 25:29-34 Now Jacob cooked a stew; and Esau came in from the field, and he *was* weary. And Esau said to Jacob, "Please feed me with that same red *stew,* for I *am* weary." Therefore his name was called Edom. But Jacob said, "Sell me your birthright as of this day." And Esau said, "Look, I *am* about to die; so what *is* this birthright to me?" Then Jacob said, "Swear to me as of this day." So he swore to him, and sold his birthright to Jacob. And Jacob gave Esau bread and stew of lentils; then he ate and drank, arose, and went his way. Thus Esau despised *his* birthright.

When you're really hungry, your body is in survival mode

You seek to remedy hunger, no matter what. If you have to ask yourself, "Am I hungry? Am I really hungry?" it is most likely not true physical hunger. Rediscovering true hunger is a process. When babies are born they eat in what has been termed *feeding on demand*. It is natural and instinctive. Because of scheduled mealtimes and activities that revolve around food and our own addictive food patterns, we have learned a different pattern of eating by instead responding to appetite and not true physical hunger.

Responding to true hunger leads to weight loss and freedom

In order to experience lasting weight loss victory and freedom, we will learn to rediscover true hunger. True hunger is not allowing anything external to prompt our eating. Eating in response to true hunger is freedom. It is natural. We can compare waiting on true hunger to a car running out of gas. We do not want to fill up the tank before it is ready for more fuel.

Fed or Fasting states

Our bodies are always in two states: ***Fed or Fasting***. During the fasting state, our bodies utilize and burn stored energy (fat), our organs rest and we usher in restoration and weight loss. God has used fasting throughout the Bible as a means of building spiritual insight and deliverance to His people. This is by no means an extended 3 day or 40 day fast. This is a state that our bodies experience everyday. When we sleep, we fast. This is the time our bodies rejuvenate and rebuild. It is called breakfast because we are *breaking the fast*.

Fasting daily for maximum wellness and weight loss

By fasting daily, while waiting on true hunger, our bodies will shed the weight more quickly. The more comfortable we become with the *fasting* state and leaving behind our unhealthy dependence on the chronic *fed* state, the more we will experience a renewed sense of energy, vitality and well-being. When we are in the fasting state, our bodies instinctively know to pull energy from our body's morbid tissue first. We are in *self-healing* mode. When we are in *fed* mode our bodies are busy digesting and metabolizing food. When we wait on hunger, we burn excess fat storage and in turn, lose weight. Once again, there is only <u>one **way**</u> to lose weight and that is to consume less and burn more. Eating by natural hunger *not* appetite or false hunger will redirect our intake to a place where we are surprisingly taking in a lot less food, feeling more energized and seeing weight loss results quickly.

The weight loss hunger response scale

Our *physical* hunger scale goes from **zero to ten**. We do not want to wait until we reach total emptiness **(zero)** because to eat in extreme hunger will provoke us to overeat.

The weight loss zone (1-5)

The best place to begin eating is around **level 1** and end around **level 5**. This is the *weight loss zone.* This is the natural zone for your body to operate. Your body's utmost wellness is attained.

A level **one** on the hunger scale is like a car almost out of gas, but you still have enough time to make it to the gas station and refuel without worrying about being stranded on the side of the road. There is no need to fear being in a place where you don't have access to food when you are hungry since our overweight bodies have excess stored energy (fat). We have, in a sense, backup fuel tanks where if we reach empty, our bodies will simply pull energy from our fat reserve. Although we encourage you to eat each time you experience hunger, we do not want you to think if you miss a meal you will die! No, most assuredly you will live.

The weight maintenance zone (5-7)

People who are uncomfortable with waiting on true hunger usually remain in the feeding zone, and typically are between **5 and 7** on the scale above. This is the *weight maintenance zone.* These are the people who are afraid to run out of gas. So as soon as they see the needle go half past full, they go to refuel. If you have been one of those people who have made statements such as, "I've always been overweight or I've always been this size." If your weight doesn't really fluctuate a lot, you probably rarely allow yourself to experience *true hunger* because you are in the habit of eating before it comes. You are what we used to call in the diet world a *grazer*. Much like cows whose eating occurs all day. We are not comfortable enough with ourselves to experience the sweet quiet comfort of *being*. God must bring us to a place where in those times of waiting for true hunger, we re-learn how to simply be and not numb the pain of our souls with food or use food and eating as a source of constant distraction.

The weight gain zone (7-10)

If you are in a cycle of your weight climbing consistently, then you are in **the weight gain zone.** You are more than likely going beyond comfortable to a place of binge eating and food abuse. You are eating between **7 and 10** on the hunger scale and inevitably you are consistently gaining weight. You are filling up your gas tank to the place where it spills over and is wasted. Your body is responding the same way. It is simply storing the excess fuel as fat, and the more you eat, the more it stores. You are the person who may be experiencing emotional pain so you numb it with your reach for food, or the person who is afraid of your own greatness so you sabotage your freedom and joy. You may even be the person who is truly afraid to let go of the instant quick fix of food to experience the lasting yet unfamiliar constant comfort of God's Holy Spirit. Through the teachings of this book, you will learn to let go of your own need to fix and manage your pain with food and wait on God's provision for your heart. You will shed the burdens on the inside and witness the power and beauty of transformation from the inside out.

Waiting on true physical hunger is the most crucial natural eating principle for lasting success

Isaiah 40:31 But those who wait on the LORD Shall renew *their* strength; They shall mount up with wings like eagles, They shall run and not be weary, They shall walk and not faint.

Your challenge to wait!

Right now, challenge yourself to wait on and respond only to true hunger. When we place our obedience to God higher than the obedience to our learned habits, His grace is ever present. It's time to break the cycle of hurting and punishing yourself with overeating. If you fall, He will pick you back up again. Eventually, you will learn His natural laws and will become consistent, relentless and focused. God is there to assist you every step of the way. It is my prayer that for the rest of this journey, you will learn how to wait on and solely respond to true hunger.

CHAPTER THREE

Overcoming Overeating

Proverbs 23:1-2 When you sit down to eat with a ruler, Consider carefully what *is* before you; And put a knife to your throat If you *are* a man given to appetite.

That scripture can sound harsh until we begin to understand the health, emotional and spiritual ramifications of overeating. If we are overweight, we are at a higher risk for a heart attack, stroke, diabetes and premature death, but more importantly spiritual death and emotional numbness. For those of us who struggle with overeating, one of our main struggles is eating past the point of comfortable satisfaction, into a place of pain. When we're in that realm, then we've crossed over into the realm of gluttony, which according to the Bible is a sin. When we eat to the point of excess, when we do not discipline our flesh and allow our spirit to govern our body, then we allow ourselves to be separated from God as we bow down to the idol of food.

Psalm 106:36 They served their idols, Which became a snare to them.

The spiritual and physical consequences of overeating

The Bible says that the wages of sin produces death (Romans 6:23). We know it is a sin to practice idolatry by placing anything or anyone higher in our hearts than God. We know that obesity- related death is second only to smoking. Smoking is the leading cause of preventable death in the United States, claiming upwards of 400,000 lives per year.

1 Peter 5:8 Be sober, be vigilant; because your adversary the devil walks about like a roaring lion, seeking whom he may devour.

Freedom from the sin of gluttony

The Bible verse says *may* which is permissive. So, I must give Satan permission to devour me, shorten my life span and wreak havoc on my physical body. I do not want to open a door to self-destruction through gluttony. When I choose to seek God's plan for renewed health, weight loss and life, I can soar to new levels of confidence and belief knowing my victory is promised in His word. We choose to focus on the Lord's plan for our lives, not our temporary fixes and band-aid cures. Jesus died on the cross to ensure we would have total and lasting freedom!

The blessing of daily self-control and surrender

I must choose to *die* to my own will *daily* in order to experience new life. God wants us to be able to exercise freedom and authority over our flesh. He desires to lead us and guide us into *all* truth. The food's comfort is temporary and so it deceives us. God's truth shows us a lasting path to restoration. In learning natural eating habits, we can lean on the strength of Christ. We can walk in the strength of Christ. We can make a daily decision, minute by minute, meal by meal to follow God's plan, be obedient to His Word and walk in gentleness and **self- control** in all things, including our eating.

Galatians 5:22-23 But the fruit of the Spirit is love, joy, peace, long-suffering, kindness, goodness, faithfulness, gentleness, self-control. Against such there is no law.

Mastering food for new freedom

It is safe to say that food makes a wonderful servant, but it promises to be a horrible master. It is not God's design that anything should master us, but rather we are more than conquerors and have the ability in Christ Jesus to overcome the dictates of our bodily appetites.

Three core natural eating principles

One: Waiting on and responding to True Physical Hunger. Eating only when you are truly physically hungry. Not from mental hunger, not from emotional hunger, not from spiritual hunger, but from true physical (stomach) hunger.

Two: Eating to the point of comfortable satisfaction. We will not gorge or stuff ourselves to the point of pain, discomfort, self-abuse or gluttony.

Three: Wise Eating. Using and exercising wisdom in my personal eating choices. Taking responsibility over my own health and food choices and eating the foods that are agreeable and favorable to my body.

Ending the cycle of overeating

We need to make a choice in our hearts that God is more important than the next bite of food. We enter this place from a place of grace, moment by moment, day by day, empowered by God's love and not our self-doubt and harsh judgment. At each and every meal, we can choose to end the cycle of overeating, self-abuse, guilt and doubt.

When is enough, enough?

One of the natural cues that help to facilitate hunger/fullness is time. Most of us eat too soon, before our bodies are physically hungry. We also eat too fast thus numbing our sensation to satisfaction and making it easier for us to move into the realm of gluttony and overeating. Once we learn to recognize the call of true physical hunger then we may soon realize that what we *think* we can eat and what our body truly *needs* can be completely different in portion size. Many nutritionists and personal trainers have adopted the principles of having their clients eat several small meals per day. This rationale is based in part on the fact that our stomach is only about the size of a large fist. Therefore, if we simply eat to accommodate the current size of our stomachs, we will eat very small portions and typically more frequently throughout the day.

The natural appetite suppressant

Our bodies desperately want to rid themselves of the excess fat and toxic storage that the overweight state produces. As we presented earlier, our bodies will *not* require food as frequently so that it may rid itself of excess weight. The same principle applies for the amount of food that I will consume in any given setting. I find it amazing when I hear stories of how shocked our workshop participants are at how little food is actually required in order for them to feel satisfied. "A half of a banana, a half of sandwich, a few bites of a burrito," and that's it, the hunger goes away. They actually feel satisfied in the physical, but the spiritual and emotional battle still wages in the mind. How can such a small amount of food satisfy me? Our focus shouldn't be on how much I can get away with eating, but how little can I eat. Remember there is only one way to lose weight and that's to *consume less* and *burn more*. Eating in response to our bodies' natural point of satisfaction is a key component to our weight loss success, and naturally reduces caloric intake.

Old habits must die for me to live

It can be painful to walk away from habits. As an overeater, I had become familiar with feeling full and stuffed after meals. Learning the discipline of leaving food on my plate and not eat everything that was served to me became an all out battle. Likewise, you may experience emotional withdrawal symptoms from the comfort that eating large portions can bring. However, you experience the hope and renewal of faith in yourself as you stop eating before becoming stuffed for renewed health and rapid weight loss..

Nothing tastes as good as freedom feels!

When the fat begins to melt off simply by your diligent response to natural eating and satisfaction signals, you will be amazed. When you daily experience the liberty of being able to say no to the last bites or leave food behind on your plate, you will know firsthand that nothing tastes as good as freedom feels!

We have the choice daily to either walk in freedom, or remain in prison; bound to the sin of gluttony. We have the opportunity daily to choose to be so full of God's Spirit, His purpose and His glory that we do not need the artificial, temporary fullness of the world's delicacies.

Eating for the right reasons

When we eat, food is simply energy. Food supplies our bodies with energy. For those of us who have extra weight to lose, then we do not require as much energy from food as a person who may be within their normal or ideal weight/size range. Our bodies will use our stored energy/fat to help us shed the pounds. Digestion takes more energy out of our body than any other function. That is why when animals are sick, they don't eat. By instinct, they know to fast and allow their bodies to utilize the energy that would be spent on digestion for healing. Likewise, when we feel sick we lose our desire to eat so that our bodies may heal, metabolize, burn morbid tissue and excess fat storage and maintain the energy necessary to restore healthy function.

Eating less to gain health and victory

In order to overcome overeating, we must choose to escape from the false belief that if we don't eat, we're going to die. Or if we don't eat, we are going to be sick. On the contrary, when we eat less, we're healthier. We feel light, energized and the weight starts to fall off and melt away. When we eat based on internal natural cues and not external habits and triggers, we're obeying God's natural plan for the body. We make a choice that allows us the freedom to move into the natural plan that God designed for our body to function optimally. God can heal and restore our mind to a place of having natural desires for food.

1 Corinthians 10:13 No temptation has overtaken you except such as is common to man; but God *is* faithful, who will not allow you to be tempted beyond what you are able, but with the temptation will also make the way of escape, that you may be able to bear *it*.

God always makes a way out of temptation

Sometimes when I'm eating and it's something that's really delicious and I have the temptation to overeat, one of my sons may call me, the phone may ring or I will hear the quiet voice of the Holy Spirit nudging me back to self-love and obedience. Something usually happens to shift my energy from the plate and once I get up, I realize that I'm not physically hungry for more.

Mastering this eating principle requires that we check in with ourselves periodically during our meal and ask ourselves, "Have I had enough?" If I listen to my body's subtle cues and quiet myself of distractions such as TV, reading and working while eating, I will find the voice of true hunger and not override its gentleness.

Cancel your "clean the plate society" membership!

Many of us grew up in a mentality that I call the "clean the plate society," where our parents taught us that we should eat everything on our plate because there were children starving in Africa, China and various other third world countries who would appreciate our food. Our parents lived by "waste not, want not." However, as adults we learn that anything we eat that is beyond the point of fullness becomes a waste in our bodies anyway.

Food goes to waste…or to your waist.

You have a trashcan in your kitchen and you have one in your body. Whatever I eat in excess that is not necessary for my body is going to waste. Toxic waste will be stored within my excess fat. At every meal, I have a choice. I can throw the rest of the food into the waste or I can put it in my system and it will not only go to my physical waistline, but it will also become toxic waste. So, either way, it's wasted.

World hunger is a poor excuse to overeat

Eating to the place of comfortable satisfaction ensures me that my body will use the food for nourishment, fuel and energy. We all hate the fact that there are children starving. However, there's something else that we can do about that besides become a glutton. We can send money to a reputable organization and/or sponsor a child in an impoverished community. But don't let the fact that there's a child starving in a third world country be an excuse for you to sit down and overeat. That is a state of mind that we must break.

Teaching our children not to overeat

When one of my three boys says, "Mommy, I'm done eating." I don't force them to clean their plates because I believe that children are born with an innate system that knows when they have had enough and when they need more. When we force our kids to clean their plates, we're developing those same habits of overeating in our children. Research shows that a child with one overweight parent has a 40% chance of becoming obese. A child with two overweight parents has an 80% chance. We cannot blame genetics, but rather we must take a closer look at the eating habits and beliefs that we are instilling within our children.

Overeating is natural...sometimes

We all have a special food that we don't get that often. Most Americans overeat at Thanksgiving. But, if we were able to eat turkey, stuffing, gravy and mashed potatoes every single day, we wouldn't overeat. Everyone feels guilty around Thanksgiving for eating to a place of discomfort, but it's simply because we don't get those special holiday foods often. The great thing about not dieting is that you don't have to finish off everything because of a fear that you won't be able to have that food again once you go back on your diet program. We have, as a society, lost the art of "special occasion eating" we stuff ourselves on delicacies daily and wonder why our waistlines are growing. A few times per year is fine...everyday is not!

The sweet freedom of delayed gratification

We can learn the discipline of delayed gratification by saving food for tomorrow. We can rest in the comfort of knowing that we can eat it later. This is actually more nurturing and more loving to make myself wait than to overburden my body, heart and digestive organs with too much food. I have to remind myself that I deserve to feel good. I am worthy of change and goodness in my life.

Eating less as a new way of life

My prayer is that when we sit down at the table to eat, we can focus on walking in love and wisdom. I pray that we would be conscious and aware of God's presence as it relates to our eating habits. There was a time when you learned how to drive a car that you had to focus on every single thing that you were doing. Now, you can drive a car while you put on lipstick, eat a cheeseburger, paint your nails and read the paper. Now let's hope you're not doing that, but most of us don't think about how we get from point A to point B, we just get there. My prayer is that eating will become such a natural process for you and when your normal weight is restored, it will just be a natural overflow of your surrender and your obedience to God.

CHAPTER FOUR

Your Body is a Temple

In the past few pages, we've learned about the power in recognizing our need for God's grace, God's power and God's strength in the struggle. Let's move from the recognition of true hunger and focus on your body being the temple of God's Holy Spirit.

1 Corinthians 6:19-20 Or do you not know that your body is the temple of the Holy Spirit *who is* in you, whom you have from God, and you are not your own? For you were bought at a price; therefore glorify God in your body and in your spirit, which are God's.

Cleaning up God's house

If you were having a very important visitor come to your house, would you clean up a little bit before they got there? Let's say Oprah Winfrey or your favorite celebrity was coming over to your house for dinner. Would you present your home in an extraordinary way for these special visitors? We have a very special visitor, who is the King of kings and the Lord of lords, and He dwells within our physical body temple every single day. Should we not present a living vessel prepared for service, healthy for action and ready to carry out God's plans on the earth? Our body is the only vehicle through which God can fulfill His purpose here on the earth. God says in His Word, "Your body is not your own. It is Mine. It was bought with a price; therefore, glorify Me in your body and in your spirit because they are Mine" (I Corinthians 6:19).

Glorifying God in our bodies

Glorify means to worship, adore, exalt, elevate and to praise. The world, on the contrary, teaches worship of the body with strict diets and extreme workout routines. They focus on worship of the physical body, but God's Word says to glorify Him in our body. We are to praise Him with our body, to honor Him with the way we treat our temple and by what we expose our bodies to.

One of the highest forms of praise is obedience. God says in His Word, "Now it shall come to pass, if you diligently obey the voice of the LORD your God, to observe carefully all His commandments which I command you today, that the LORD your God will set you high above all nations of the earth" (Deuteronomy 28:1).

There is no separation between body and spirit

When we are walking in obedience to God's plan for our temples, our actions become our daily acts of worship. The Bible says to glorify God in our body and our spirit, which is God's. There's no separation between body and spirit; God wants us to surrender them both. It is a popular secular mentality to think "what I do with *my* body is what I do with *my* body." But there was a price paid on Calvary for *my* body, *my* redemption and *my* salvation. When I decide to die to my own will and seek new life in Christ, the actions I make in this body become an active, powerful part of my worship.

Romans 12:1 I beseech you therefore, brethren, by the mercies of God, that you present your bodies a living sacrifice, holy, acceptable to God, *which is* your reasonable service.

Giving God your body daily

When I compare the mercies of God and the ultimate sacrifice on the cross of Jesus Christ, isn't it just reasonable that I would sacrifice my body to Him daily? Paul is saying that it is a reasonable act of service for us to give up our bodies as a living sacrifice in light of God's mercy. The word reasonable means practical, sound or rational. It's just rational that, in light of what Jesus Christ did for me, I would wake up every morning and say, "Lord, I give you my body today."

Natural change through a surrendered heart

A surrendered heart will make it so much easier for you to push away from the plate, for you to get up off of the couch, for you to walk around the block. God transforms the heart first and the body follows. He does a marvelous work from the inside out. Man focuses on the *outer weight*. God changes the heart and releases us from the *inner-weights* and burdens that have fueled the cycle of our addictions. Glorifying God in my physical body means to magnify Him, to make Him big and make me small. We so often do the opposite. We make ourselves, our food struggles and our weight large, and make God small.

John 3:30 He must increase, but I *must* decrease.

When we magnify God and make Him large in every single situation in our lives, we won't have the need to run to food out of a fear of failure. God will become so big in our lives and the fact of the matter is the bigger we allow Him to become, the smaller our problems and bodies become.

2 Corinthians 4:18 While we do not look at the things which are seen, but at the things which are not seen. For the things which are seen *are* temporary, but the things which are not seen *are* eternal.

Do I want a quick diet fix? Or do I desire lasting freedom?

Do I want a quick prescription drug fix or do I want permanent healing? When we choose to focus on something that has value in this life and in the life to come, we begin the healing work by daily honoring Christ, knowing that only what we do for Christ will last. We are eager for the *product*, but God is interested in the *process*. It is the *process* that teaches and empowers us with the necessary tools to maintain and excel in our desired vision.

A new temple vision

When we put God first, our physical temple is going to reveal the manifestation of that choice. It will no longer look like a temple built through pain, shame, disappointment and fear. It will begin to shape itself and look like a temple built by His love, His promise, His mercy and His grace. So when the world looks at me, they will see a woman who looks like she's in love with her Maker.

Are you in love or pain?

When you see a woman in love, she looks like a woman in love. When you see a man in pain, he looks like a man in pain. We focus on the inside principle of stewardship over God's property. We focus on the internal, eternal principle of worshipping God with our physical temple and therein lies our victory. Although these are spiritual concepts, we will witness physical wellness, weight loss, vitality and energy restored in the natural. When we put the focus on Christ and not self, the constant struggle will cease.

Love will empower my daily actions that produce weight loss

The commitment to daily honor God in our treatment and care of our body temple is one that we must fight to uphold. God is more focused on who we are *being* than what we are *doing*. When our hearts are fully surrendered to His Will, when we truly love Him with all of our soul, strength and entire mind, then taking care of this temple and standing on His promises becomes a natural by-product of the love that we have for Him. Love is action, not mere words. I show my love for a most gracious God through my daily walk.

Deuteronomy 10:12 And now, Israel, what does the LORD your God require of you, but to fear the LORD your God, to walk in all His ways and to love Him, to serve the LORD your God with all your heart and with all your soul.

CHAPTER FIVE

Wise Eating

Exodus 3:17 and I have said I will bring you up out of the affliction of Egypt to the land of the Canaanites and the Hittites and the Amorites and the Perizzites and the Hivites and the Jebusites, to a land flowing with milk and honey.

Was that low fat milk Lord and reduced-calorie honey?

Much like the Israelites, who had been prisoners of the Egyptians, many of us have been prisoners to a system of thought and have been living a life of bondage to our bodies. Our all-consuming thoughts of food, fat and dieting have created a prison *within*. When God led His people out of captivity, He promised to bring them into a land flowing with His abundance, goodness and provision. We will find that when we seek God, our eating will be more enjoyable. God made food and it is good. I love a good piece of dark chocolate, a fresh bowl of strawberries, a homemade bowl of hot, chicken tortilla soup with crispy, Mexican, corn tortilla chips and spicy salsa or a fresh, homemade, juicy burger with all the trimmings. I thoroughly enjoy most foods in moderation. God has put so many bountiful foods here for our enjoyment and given us dominion and authority over everything. Food is not the problem, overeating is. When I make food *neutral*, I remove its power and my need to rebel and overeat.

Proverbs 2:6 For the LORD gives wisdom; From His mouth *come* knowledge and understanding

Wise eating produces weight loss and wellness

We make over 2,000 choices every single day. How do we know what God would have us to do? Deciding when, how much and what to eat will now be based on careful attention to our needs and God's wisdom working in us, not the outer dictates of a diet. A lot of diet programs and commercial diet centers will tell us that we need to eat a certain amount of food, at certain times and in certain combinations. When we consider that different people have different energy levels, nutritional needs, bio-chemical make-up, intake requirements, physical activity levels and digestive responses to food, it doesn't make sense that two people should follow the same meal plan. For one person, it may be adequate. For another person, it may not fulfill their energy requirements. Trying to stick to a meal plan can set a person up for overeating as well as the many physical and emotional effects of restricting food. It's been estimated that there are more than *26,000* different diets in the world. They all have a concept on how *they* think *we* should eat and yet each year, the obesity population in America continues to soar along with sickness and poor health. There are even countless Biblical approaches to weight loss that all take their different points of view on how we should eat.

Taking personal responsibility for my own eating habits

We teach in our Body Temple Wellness workshops that true healing starts when everyone seeks their own truth. It's easy to point the blame at a diet principle or program and say, "I tried it and it didn't work." It's another thing to pursue God and develop your own convictions and wisdom as it relates to the health of your body and your family. In order to walk in renewed health and well-being in every aspect of our lives, we must seek wisdom. Just like every other principle we teach, your new eating habits will begin from the inside out. Diets focus on food management, yet it is temporary and in most cases never produces permanent life change. Most people who eat from a standpoint of personal convictions make food choices that mirror their beliefs. In order to develop a lifestyle that does not make food the enemy, we must examine our hearts and seek God's wisdom in regards to our personal eating.

Dieting is "serving" food

Dieting to lose weight makes us a servant to food through complicated menus, food combinations, measuring, weighing and counting carbs and calories. We are to master food, not serve it. When you eat from a place of wisdom, food becomes your servant and not your master.

Proverbs 4:20-22 My son, give attention to my words; Incline your ear to my sayings. Do not let them depart from your eyes; Keep them in the midst of your heart; For they *are* life to those who find them, And health to all their flesh. This scripture speaks of the importance of wisdom. The words of wisdom can bring life for those who seek them and health to a man's entire body. In order to walk in the fullness of what God intends for us, we must stop looking to the world for answers. The world and unbelievers should look to us as we seek God and are led into truth. The Bible says that "we are the light of the world" (Matthew 5:14). We should illuminate truth in areas where there is darkness, confusion and lack of understanding.

Wisdom in not following the world's failing methods

The diet world has built a 40 billion dollar business on the premise of failure. The fact that statistics show that 97-99% of dieters fail at long-term weight loss success is proof that the industry continues to thrive as we continue to fail. God can use His people to bring truth to a dying world and allow the power of God to demonstrate healing, wellness and lasting weight loss through a personal relationship with Jesus Christ. At our Body Temple Wellness workshops, we do not provide participants with a list of do's and don'ts in regards to their eating choices. We understand that the diet world is failing us with similar lists. One year, carbs are good and the next year, they are bad. One year, it's high protein and the next year, we're all vegan. We have been seeking the world and leaning on our own understanding in regards to health. Instead, we should seek the Divine Creator who made our marvelous bodies.

Proverbs 3:5-6 Trust in the LORD with all your heart, And lean not on your own understanding; In all your ways acknowledge Him, And He shall direct your paths.

God is the master craftsman behind our bodies and our lives.

He gave us a marvelous body. Here are a few facts that you may not know about how gloriously God fashioned our temples. Your body houses 10 different organ systems, nearly 700 muscles, 206 bones, 2 kidneys and a heart that beats involuntarily 100,000 times per day, over 3 billion times for the average lifespan. There is a liver that is responsible for 500 different functions in our body. There are nearly 45 miles of nerves funneling through your body. Each person has a unique tongue print that contains about 10,000 taste buds and no two finger prints are alike. In one square inch of skin lie 4 yards of nerve fibers, 1300 nerve cells, 100 sweat glands, 3 million cells, and 3 yards of blood vessels. We have a complex digestive system/tract that consists of an intricate tube more than 30 feet long that is lined with a mucous membrane. With the exception of your brain cells, 50 million of the cells in your body will have died and been replaced with new ones in the short amount of time it took for you to finish reading this sentence!

God has a personalized plan for my success!

God's creation is a masterpiece that has inspired and baffled the minds of scientists for hundreds of years. After countless billions have been spent on medical research, much about the human body in relationship to disease, health and even weight loss still confounds the limitations of modern medicine and science-based data. This body, this physical vessel, is God's tool to accomplish His plan in our lives while we are on earth. Who better to seek for health and understanding than the God who formed us in our mother's womb?

Jeremiah 1:5 Before I formed you in the womb I knew you; Before you were born I sanctified you; I ordained you a prophet to the nations.

God knows our genetic makeup, our chemical imbalances, our predispositions and our weaknesses in regards to our eating habits. Who better to seek for wisdom and understanding than the God who promises to lead us to victory?!

Proverbs 4:3-6 When I was my father's son, tender and the only one in the sight of my mother, He also taught me, and said to me: "Let your heart retain my words; Keep my commands, and live. Get wisdom! Get understanding! Do not forget, nor turn away from the words of my mouth. Do not forsake her, and she will preserve you; Love her, and she will keep you."

A calorie is a calorie

God gave us food for our enjoyment. We understand that, in a very simple sense, a calorie is a calorie, or unit of energy. Our bodies use calories for one thing...survival. The energy we get from food keeps our heart beating, blood pumping to our organs and our lungs pumping oxygen through breathing. Calories keep your internal organs operating properly. They keep the brain running properly and efficiently. They keep our body warm and give us the fuel to accomplish our daily tasks. When we eat or consume calories, our bodies use or burn the calories through a complex series of metabolic processes, in which digestive enzymes break down the carbohydrates, fats and proteins into molecules such as glucose, fatty acids and amino acids. These are then transported through the blood stream to our cells where they are either absorbed (used) immediately or stored. In the most basic sense, our bodies will use the energy they need and store the rest as fat.

No more diet games!

Diets have taught us to manipulate and lower our caloric intake, sometimes even drastically, to capitalize on the only true weight loss principle. *Eat less, burn more.* However, when we succumb to an unrealistic way of life that teaches us to glory in the outer appearance of momentary food management and behavior modification, we set ourselves up for failure. It is only a matter of time before we go back to our normal way of eating and gain the weight that we lost and, in most cases, a few more pounds. If you have ever played the "diet game" before, then you know that it is just that…a game. We can keep up the activity for a period of time until we reach our "goal" but to keep the weight off is a different story. A story, more often than not, that ends in disappointment and discouragement. We fail to realize that we have to do exactly what we did to get the weight off in order to maintain our new physique.

Can you diet for the rest of your life?

We must be honest in our evaluations of the rest of our lives. Can we honestly live with a juice fast or cabbage soup or only raw foods or even no carbs, bread or potatoes for the rest of our earthly life? It is a personal choice, but most of us do not look at the long-term bigger picture. We know that true lasting change begins in the heart. For those who are seeking momentary weight changes only to regain what was lost, then a diet is a safe and possibly familiar choice. For those who are seeking life change, permanent weight loss and freedom, Jesus is the way, the truth and the light!

Our lives are a sum total of the choices that we have made

God's wisdom is practical and will manifest itself in a tangible sense through our daily actions and choices. When people observe our lives, they witness wisdom or in some cases, foolishness. God instructs us in Luke 14:28 to "count the cost" for the decisions we make and the plans we declare in our hearts. And as we approach weight loss and wellness from the inside-out, we must count the cost of what we are willing to do differently to gain a different result.

1 Corinthians 6:12-13 All things are lawful for me, but all things are not helpful. All things are lawful for me, but I will not be brought under the power of any. Foods for the stomach and the stomach for foods, but God will destroy both it and them. Now the body *is* not for sexual immorality but for the Lord, and the Lord for the body.

Taking ownership over my eating choices

We believe that all food is good food and that God wants us to enjoy the blessings of His abundance. We are in a land that overflows with milk and honey. Guilt is produced by the diet mentality of "good" and "bad" food choices. That destructive emotion of guilt and shame only causes me to overeat when I'm "off" my program and then I obsess over the foods that I cannot have when I am dieting. If we take the focus off of the distraction of food, we are forced to look where many of us have not wanted to all along…at our own hearts, pain and fear. We must realize that food is neutral and that the choices we make should be born from ownership of our eating habits and not dictated by the latest diet guru or miracle cure weight loss plan.

Eating the foods that are right for my body

Wisdom is paying attention and nurturing our own needs and realize that while all food is *permissible,* not all food is *beneficial* for our personal bodies, including some foods pushed by popular diets. For instance, let's say you are a person with a family history of kidney problems and you follow the masses and enter a high-protein diet, not knowing that years later you would pay for that temporary weight loss by way of renal/kidney failure. This is because high-protein diets are very taxing to our kidneys and other organs. In the past, before I permanently lost my weight with the methods outlined in this book, I tried many diets where the focus was high dairy intake, cheese, non-fat yogurt and cottage cheese. Well, I am lactose intolerant. So, following in these sorts of diets left me with minimal weight loss but plenty of bloating and gas. We must *know* our own bodies. When we seek God's wisdom and study our own family history, we make choices that add to our longevity and produce weight loss at the same time.

Food for health and wellness, not just weight loss

We must look past temporary weight loss to a higher level of health and understanding. We should be at a place where we are maturing past the image of that size 6 dress size and instead focus on the image and vision of health, longevity, wellness, energy, confidence and strength! Food plays a role in how we feel and it is our personal responsibility to eat the foods that benefit our personal body. Each one of us has a different chemical makeup. Each of our bodies is designed differently. That is by design that not even two fingerprints are the same. That is why I have a hard time in my field with people who proclaim their way as "the only way" to weight loss, the miracle cure of scientific truth. There is nothing wrong with seeking wise counsel and understanding in regards to your personal eating choices.

Proverbs 19:20 Listen to counsel and receive instruction, that you may be wise in your latter days.

Sure, I believe that God gives vision and understanding to men so that they may be a blessing to creation, but I think it is pretty arrogant to say that my way is the only way to weight loss or wellness when clearly our paths, just like our fingerprints, will be different. We must make it our business to know, learn about and commit to our personal path. What your own heart believes and is convicted by is what you will commit to. The changes in your eating will start and end with you, not anything outside of you. It's time to take ownership and responsibility for your eating.

My personal standards for food...

I have a standard on what neighborhood I would want to raise my children. I have a standard when it comes to the quality of music I listen to, the programs I watch on TV, the people I would partner with in vision, the skin and hair care products I use, the detergent I use and the diapers I put on my babies. So, you better believe that I will have standards when it comes to the fuel I put in my body to sustain my life. And likewise, we all should have our own set of standards and convictions in regards to our choices. I know that there are certain things that I cannot eat, certain foods that just don't agree with me. The Holy Spirit says that He will lead you and "guide you into all truth" (John 16:13). I believe that means everything including our food choices. During the process of learning our bodies, we can go directly to the source and request that God would direct our path into this new life and body we are seeking.

Eating choices rooted in wisdom, rooted in love

My personal eating choices have nothing to do with a "diet mentality", nor were any of my food convictions motivated through a fear-based thinking of fat loss or weight gain. I know that I can lose or gain weight pretty much on any given food. Weight is lost one way, by using more energy than I take in. It's that plain and simple. My choices are motivated by self-love, respect for my husband, children and the legacy of health I wish to leave to my future generations. My choices are motivated out of reverence for God in the way I treat this masterpiece that He has created. I encourage you to develop your own list of personal eating convictions.

Love and Wisdom requires saying "no" in my eating habits

Another practice in wise eating is not allowing myself something simply because I *want* it but truly asking myself do I *need* it? One of the greatest words we can tell ourselves is *no* when we know the choice we are making will not aid us in achieving our vision of a new body and restored health. Decision making is actually quite simple once your vision is clear. If the choice moves you closer to your goal, the answer is "yes" if it does not, the answer is "no." The entitlement, pleasure-seeking mentality is what has created the cycle of poor discipline and discernment in regards to our eating. I am making a choice to change now. It is important to make consistent decisions in regards to habits that will keep me in a place of wellness and weight loss.

Becoming an expert about my own body

As dieters, we want somebody to just show us the plan. "Tell me what to eat. Tell me when to eat. Tell me how much I should eat." We shift all the responsibility to the man holding the diet book. We shift all the responsibility to the latest doctor who's come out with a new scientific method for us to lose weight, when God gives us wisdom to become experts on our own bodies. I consider myself to be an expert in my own health. Most times, I know immediately when a particular food does not "sit right with me." Most people turn to pills, laxatives and antacids to give band-aid cures to their food problems, but we can choose to eat foods that make us feel good and benefit our lifestyle. When we truly enter a place of self-love and respect, we will be mindful of what we eat and how it affects our lives. As we embrace and adopt new *Spirit led* habits, we will be willing to let the *lesser* things die such as our cravings, addictions and habits. It is then that the *greater* may live, our legacy, inheritance and health.

As I decrease, He will increase

I believe that each one of us has something that we're holding on to or something that's a part of our lifestyle, our habitual eating that God may call us to surrender or release to Him. Seek His face and be willing to give up the parts of your lifestyle where you have become a slave to food and the indulgences of the flesh.

Becoming a wise eater

It's time to take ownership over our personal eating choices. We should make it a habit to pay attention to the way we feel 30 minutes to an hour after we eat. "Do I have energy? Do I feel lethargic? Do I feel tired? Do I feel groggy? Do I feel bloated, heart burn or upset stomach?" These are not signs to ignore or medicate. This is our body's way of letting us know what foods, portions and combinations of food are not *beneficial* for us. We live in a society that teaches us to take drugs, like antacids, when we feel heartburn or indigestion. Drugs only mask the cry of our body. If we continually abuse our systems with the same foods that cause us discomfort, we are not practicing wisdom in our eating habits.

Food for energy and longevity

Pay attention to your body. Treat it like a temple and do not allow anything to defile your body. Use wisdom when you eat and make it a practice to study and learn your own system. We want to move into a consistent lifestyle that uses food not only for pleasure and enjoyment, but also energy and longevity. When we finish eating, we should get up feeling light, energetic and excited, because food is energy. And if we are in a place where the energy or fuel that we're putting into our systems does not agree with our system, then it's not the right kind of fuel for us.

Wise eating is for freedom, not diet-based legalism

Colossians 2:21-23 "Do not touch, do not taste, do not handle," which all concern things which perish with the using—according to the commandments and doctrines of men? These things indeed have an appearance of wisdom in self-imposed religion, *false* humility, and neglect of the body, *but are* of no value against the indulgence of the flesh.

People can make a religion of how they eat. These outside regulations have nothing to do with the indulgence of the flesh. The main focus with us is a matter of our spirit. It's not about the calories. It's not just about the food that's on the plate. It's about the heart.

Biblical food legalism is still a diet!

Many new Biblical-based weight loss programs offer this same sort of legalism, encouraging people to only eat like the people in the Old Testament. However, the Old Testament food restrictions were rendered null and void when Jesus declared that His covenant was better than one based on the law. The law proved one thing to man...that He was incapable of keeping it. In Christ, we find grace to bring us into a place of mastery over the flesh, a mastery and freedom that restrictive diets and food management could never offer. In Jesus, we have *the inner cleansing* by His blood; therefore we do not have to live by rigid *outer cleanliness* in regards to our food. There is truth and wisdom in the Old Testament law of God and that may be the very place you are led to gain knowledge for your personal eating habits. But let that be your personal choice. A choice that you are willing to follow and stick to from a place of faith and conviction, not temporary aims at weight loss.

Jesus: the traveling food connoisseur

Jesus for much of His ministry did not have a home. He went from house to house and also instructed His disciples to "eat whatever was set before them" (Luke 10:8). Although I'm sure that he wasn't being offered fried chicken or chili cheese burgers, His focus was always centered on what was in the heart of man, not what he was putting in his mouth.

When God is first, my eating habits will change for the better

In Christ, there's a deeper level that we can go to, where we're not focused on all the foods that we are manipulating on the outside. Instead, we can get to a place of true surrender where there is nothing in this world that we value higher than God. Personally, I so earnestly want to honor Him in the way I treat my body...which is

His temple that I am willing to allow transformation in the way I eat and view food. When I practice wise eating, I am eating, in a sense, by faith. God becomes first place in my life, not food.

Corinthians 10:31 Therefore, whether you eat or drink, or whatever you do, do all to the glory of God.

My steps become ordered by His Word and not by my appetites, cravings and addictions. When our eating is fully surrendered to the wisdom of Christ, we will witness the lasting, supernatural and natural changes in our life and body. We will relish in the freedom, liberty and victory promised to us in Christ.

CHAPTER SIX

How Faith Changes Shape

With our 200 plus channels, wide-screen TV's, cell phones, e-mail and all of the technology that is supposed to enhance our pleasure and free time, we have become culprits of the couch potato syndrome; leading sedentary lifestyles. Countless medical research documents that leading a sedentary lifestyle has a huge effect on our health as well as our emotional, physical, mental and spiritual well-being. I know that with the diet mentality, there comes a focus on extreme exercise. "Oh, if I just exercise, I would lose weight." Beyond using exercise for momentary weight loss efforts, God calls those of us who are physically able to a level of diligent practice and self-mastery.

We master our bodies and not allow our bodies to master us.

We've all started exercise regimens before, but it is estimated that less than 15% of adults in America get the recommended daily amount of physical movement necessary. Why? Do you really want to become focused and consistent with your physical activity? Then let's approach it from a higher level, let's approach fitness from the spirit first. When we allow God's Word to transform our minds, our actions will change and become consistent with His wisdom for our bodies. We are not to be lazy, slothful or a sluggard, but earnest in our desire to please God in every area of our lives.

Moving my body benefits mind, body and spirit

From a spiritual perspective, we move and desire fitness because we want to bring this flesh into submission. There's a physical aspect to it as far as how we feel – our energy. We also decrease our risk for so many diseases. There's an emotional aspect to it because exercise has been linked to better mental health, lower depression, anxiety and fatigue. And just like Esther in the Bible, who submitted to a strict regime of purification, beauty treatments, diet and exercise, we will look better, become fabulously fit and fine! We do not approach exercise from the "diet mentality" that screams, "If I don't work out, I'll be fat forever!" But rather, we approach it from a mature level of exercising for our body, mind and spirit that is born out of a need, a necessity and a desire to please God in all things – not just to lose weight. We approach it to feel better, to love and nurture our bodies and to walk in wholeness and wellness.

Was Jesus a couch potato?

Jesus was not a lazy or slothful person. He was so much about purpose, so much about the will of the Father that I believe His lifestyle was one of being active and involved. Biblical scholars, who have traced the steps of Jesus over His three year ministry, have estimated that He walked upwards of 18,000 miles! That breaks down to 16 miles per day. 16 miles for purpose, passion and to accomplish the will of the Father! I believe that the disciples as well as the early church were the same way because walking was a part of their daily lifestyle. To get their food and to wash their clothes, there was physical labor involved in every aspect of life. The early church did not deal with the amount of obesity and sickness that comes from leading an inactive lifestyle. There was a famous phase that asked the question, *What would Jesus do?* Well apparently, Jesus would walk!

Proverbs 13:4 The soul of a lazy *man* desires, and *has* nothing; But the soul of the diligent shall be made rich.

I compare the lazy man's soul, who desires and gets nothing, to a person who watches infomercials. Many infomercials promise five-minute fitness, two-minute abs and 6-day miracle diets! They're appealing to the soul of the lazy man. And with all of our modern infomercials, which are a large part of the 40 billion dollar diet industry, we remain the most sedentary, obese and inactive industrialized nation in the entire world. The Body of Christ should look different from an inactive, complacent, entertainment and pleasure-seeking world. Faith is action, so when people look at our lives they should witness movement and consistent improvement!

Consistency is the key to victory!

We shovel billions of dollars each year into an industry that promises us a quick fix when it's our soul that needs transformation. Life is not a quick fix. You cannot microwave or make instant lasting results. Life change comes through diligence. We look for the big-bang or the latest breakthrough, but true change comes from the small day to day decisions that we make. Weight loss and wellness victory are directly tied to consistency. I used to work with a personal trainer at Body Temple Wellness and women would constantly come up to her and say, "Oh, I wish I had a body like yours. You're so lucky." And she would say, "I'm not lucky. This is 16 years of diligence in my life that you see standing before you. This is not something that I stumbled into. This body is by design."

Does your walk match your talk?

Many of us desire a different body and renewed health. But the scripture says that the lazy man desires and has nothing. In the original text the biblical word *belief* meant the same as the word *do*. What you *believe* or confess with your mouth, people should be able to see or witness you *do*. It takes diligence to sustain health and wealth. True change occurs when we demonstrate an active willingness to submit our bodies and minds to God's Word on a daily basis. True change comes when we *do* what we *say* we desire.

Ecclesiastes 10:17 Blessed *are* you, O land, when your king *is* the son of nobles, And your princes feast at the proper time— For strength and not for drunkenness!

The value of discipline and self-control

Food is supposed to be our energy but overeating causes it to actually rob us of energy. When we eat to the point of drunkenness, we have no desire to move our bodies. We are led by our feelings and emotions instead of governing our body through the strength of the Holy Spirit and self-control. We have long admired athletes and tri-athletes, Iron Men and fierce competitors. We see in them a level of discipline and diligence to be esteemed. God is calling us to be champions as well, to live our best life as far as our energy, our health and our well being. All of those things are impacted by physical activity.

Ecclesiastes 10:18 Because of laziness the building decays, and through idleness of hands the house leaks.

Inactivity carries a heavy price tag

When we don't take care of our bodies, things start to decay. Things start to break down. We can look at this physical house and see how it's torn down and it decays. Our lifespan, muscles, energy, health, moods and overall quality of life can be severely impacted. People fail to realize that when they choose to do nothing, they are actually doing something powerful indeed. Inactivity and the failure to move bears heavier consequences than most people care to own. As we age, we can experience fatigue from imbalances in our bodies such as arthritis, lower back problems or other ailments that effect mobility. As these conditions grow progressively worse, many people adopt the false mentality that if they rest, they will get better. On the contrary, when we become inactive, we feel more fatigued and tired because our choice not to move has decreased our overall physical fitness. It begets a vicious cycle. Disability and body aches feed into a sedentary lifestyle and a sedentary life and inactivity results in higher levels of bodily dysfunction.

Lack of movement can sabotage our future independence

Over a period of time, our choice to not move may result in a quality of life where we are dependent upon on the help of people and medical equipment to assist with the normal activities of daily life such as climbing stairs, bathing, walking or doing household chores. The more we use our bodies, the stronger they become, the healthier we become and the longer we live with strength and vitality. In certain cultures, such as Japan and Italy or in religious groups such as Seventh-Day Adventists and Mormons, you have people living and enjoying their body for the miracle that it is in their 70's, 80's or even 100's. People of these ages are running, riding bikes, swimming or even climbing up a mountainside!

How does physical movement and exercise affect our health?

- Reduces the risk of dying prematurely from heart disease.
- Reduces the risk of developing diabetes.
- Reduces the risk of developing high blood pressure.
- Helps reduce blood pressure in people who already have high blood pressure.
- Reduces the risk of developing colon cancer.
- Reduces feelings of depression and anxiety.
- Helps control weight.
- Helps build and maintain healthy bones, muscles and joints.
- Helps older adults become stronger and better able to move around without falling.
- Promotes psychological well-being.

Deuteronomy 34:7 Moses *was* one hundred and twenty years old when he died. His eyes were not dim nor his natural vigor diminished.

In our modern society, we expect our bodies to wear out and breakdown with age. We see aches, pains and sickness as normal aspects of aging, yet time and time again in the Bible, we are presented with the stories of those who lived well into their hundreds. Moses incorporated the world's most inexpensive and most effective form of exercise...he walked! The 40 years that he spent with the children of Israel in the desert was not in a SUV, it was on foot.

The easiest and most natural exercise around!

They walked day in and day out and their bodies were stronger because of their movement. We neglect this truly wonderful form of exercise. It sounds and looks easy, but most of us do not bother to walk. Instead, we prefer to sign up for expensive aerobic classes or fool ourselves into thinking we can only get fit in a gym. Where were gyms a hundred years ago? Where were they in Biblical times? People used their natural environment for fitness. Fresh air, greenery and natural surroundings surpass the closed-in walls and man-made machines of a gym. I am not saying to not use the gym as a part of your personal fitness quest. I use my local gym for their lap-pool and basketball court. What I am saying is don't let not making it to the gym be the excuse you offer for inactivity. The only equipment that you need to walk is a pair of tennis shoes.

Walking adds strength where we need it most

Muscle strength and endurance is needed to complete activities of daily living. If you want to live a life independent of the constant assistance of others, then walking can have a major impact on your physical endurance and muscle strength. You don't even have to add weights to your walking because the mere act engages our muscles. We build them just by walking. The more muscles your body has, the more stored energy/fat you will burn. When you focus on adhering to the natural eating principles outlined in this book, you will eat less. When you incorporate a muscle strengthening activity such as walking, even when you are resting, your body will burn more energy/calories if it contains more muscle. Experts believe that muscle strength and endurance are the most important components of physical fitness for older adults. Research has shown that there is a significant loss in muscle strength starting at age 45, continuing to age 65 and further declines in the seventh and eighth decades of life. When we daily engage our bodies through walking, like great Biblical leaders before us, we do not have to become weak and worn out with age.

Joshua 14:10-11 And now, behold, the LORD has kept me alive, as He said, these forty-five years, ever since the LORD spoke this word to Moses while Israel wandered in the wilderness; and now, here I am this day, eighty-five years old. As yet I *am as* strong this day as on the day that Moses sent me; just as my strength *was* then, so now *is* my strength for war, both for going out and for coming in.

Getting stronger with age.

Heart disease is the number one killer of Americans. It is the number one killer of women. As women, we often feel guilty about doing things for ourselves. This is the one activity where we cannot afford to sit still, for the sake of our loved ones. Keeping our hearts strong through walking can keep us strong. Caleb was as strong as he was at *eighty five as he was at forty five.* That is an awesome testimony for strength and endurance. Recently my best friend's grandmother suffered a stroke at 89 years old. Before the stroke, she walked three miles a day every morning for over 20 years. Her recovery was so swift, her doctors all raved about how quickly she regained mobility on both sides of her body. Her physical therapist knew that her walking regimen played a major role in her rapid recovery. Everyday that she walked, she was investing in an account that she would later need to withdraw from. Witnessing her remarkable recovery proved that her investment truly paid off!

Moving beyond the diet mentality

It's time for us to move from the diet mentality of seeing exercise as a tool for quick weight loss and approach it from a standpoint of saving and prolonging our lives. When we walk every day, for at least 30 minutes, we keep our circulatory system in good condition. This system consists of our heart, blood vessels and lungs. Research has consistently proven that good cardiovascular endurance decreases our risks for high cholesterol, high blood pressure, stroke and heart attack.

Are you too busy to live longer?

In spite of all these awesome benefits that physical fitness brings to our lives and health, we don't do it. The number one reason people claim not to be able to exercise is time. God ministered to my spirit recently that if I am too busy to exercise then *I am just plain too busy*. Because exercise builds strength in our cardiovascular system, we will have tremendous amounts of energy to accomplish our daily tasks when we put first things first. The great thing about walking is there really is no excuse, with the exception of bad weather. We can increase our walking everyday in real life situations such as running errands, parking further from the store, as well as focused walking just for fitness. Walking is sowing a seed into our life-span and aiding our body's natural defense against disease and chronic illness.

Titus 1:12 One of them, a prophet of their own, said, "Cretans *are* always liars, evil beasts, lazy gluttons."

Whenever the Bible speaks of a lazy person, it does not speak of them in a positive light. There are times that the word lazy is tied into the fact that our eating habits are not in line with how the Lord wants them to be. Gluttony is excess. So, in one area of our lives, we're excessive, lazy, physically inactive and extremely out of balance. This is a recipe for poor health, lack of confidence and depression. Continuing in this cycle can wreak havoc on our bodies, emotions and spiritual life.

1 Corinthians 9:26-27 Therefore I run thus: not with uncertainty. Thus I fight: not as one who beats the air. But I discipline my body and bring *it* into subjection, lest, when I have preached to others, I myself should become disqualified.

Paul talks about how our bodies need to be our servant and not our master. Many of us lead lives from the opposite direction – we're led by our feelings. We are actually servants to our feelings, our bodies and food instead of masters. I believe that God gives us the strength in Christ to be a master over this physical body, emotions and appetites. We can chose daily action liberated from the shackles of excuse-making.

Entertain me to death...

Studies have shown that we as Christians are more overweight than any other organized religious group. The African American community actually exceeds the average rates for high blood pressure, heart attack, stroke and renal (kidney) failure. What happened to God's great and mighty people? They all got cable and wide-screen TV's. Did we get so comfortable in a place of being entertained, that we are entertaining ourselves to death? We make it a point in our home not to watch a lot of television. Not only have studies proven that excessive television watching is directly tied into the sedentary lifestyle, but it is also linked with depression and low mood. As God's people, we can enjoy entertainment, but when it gets to the place where I am spending more free time watching somebody else's life rather than designing my own, I have failed to realize my full potential in Christ and His marvelous plan for my life.

A yielded vessel is a moving vessel

God said in His Word that "for everyone to whom much is given, from him much will be required" (Luke 12:48). I serve Him with all of me, including my body. When I am in a posture of praise and honor, I am a yielded vessel willing to share the gospel or walk around the block. As Christians, we are called to be a peculiar people. We are to stand out and look different, lead by example. If my lifestyle of chronic inactivity mirrors the world, then something must change...me.

Proverbs 21:25 The desire of the lazy *man* kills him, for his hands refuse to labor.

Sick, fat and death by grace...

We have adopted a mentality in the church that sounds a little weird to the world and rightfully so. We expect to live however we want to live, do whatever we want to do. We say a quick prayer, attend a Sunday healing service to get hands laid on us and in Jesus' name, everything will be just fine! After all, we are *saved by grace!* I believe in the supernatural healing power of God. I believe God is very much in the miracle business. I also think it is fair to say that we have a mentality which borderlines on arrogance when we think we are not subject to natural laws. If you jump off of a building, you will die or severely injure yourself. That is the law of gravity. Even Jesus said we are not to *tempt God* when it comes to natural laws (Matthew 4:7). We have natural laws in regards to our bodies. Everything about our bodies tells us that they were made for movement. With our desk jobs and internet-driven lifestyles, we do not get the amount of natural movement that other cultures do and we are paying for it big time.

We are subject to natural laws for health and wellness

In the church, we put so much emphasis on the "big sins" and miss that God wants us to have discipline over this physical vessel because discipline and obedience will spill into so many other areas of our lives. For when we operate by God's natural laws, we experience the best that life has to offer. We see a power working within our own lives that causes us to rise to the occasion of greatness without fear.

I must take personal responsibility for the quality of my life

When we engage our bodies in physical activity, we take advantage of natural laws that increase our longevity and quality of life. We can stop using excuses like "when it's my time to go, it's just my time" and "Oh well, everybody's going to die some day!" This way of thought gives us the excuse to not take ownership and responsibility over the quality of our own lives. We know that the Bible says faith without works is dead (James 2:14). Likewise, if we proclaim Christ is the center of our weight loss and wellness plan, then that should take on the form of daily actions to move us closer toward our victory and new life.

Jesus walked, and so will we

If you would like to join the women and men in the Body Temple Wellness workshops, who have committed to a lifestyle of walking, we invite you to join us! Here are some simple steps to follow below. Many of our members have decided to join the 10,000 steps a day campaign, aimed at a lifestyle of fitness. Participants agree to 10,000 steps per day recorded by a pedometer or a step counter that they wear at all waking hours. This can include an organized, purposeful, fitness walk. However, the 10,000 step belief encourages us to be mindful of increasing our activity (steps) around the home, work and play. These steps average about 4.5 miles a day. This may sound like a lot, but most active New Yorkers walk this much everyday just as a part of their lifestyle. Also remember, it is estimated that Jesus may have walked upwards of 16 miles per day. That is over 35,000 steps per day. We highly encourage 10,000 steps per day.

Why 10,000 steps?

This system for lifestyle fitness has proven to be quite effective because it gives people measurable goals that they can track and monitor throughout the day. When you make it a habit to wear a pedometer or step counter, you are making a choice to challenge yourself to live an active life. It is sometimes easier to track your personal progress when you have an awesome motivational tool such as a pedometer to remind you of how many or how little steps you have taken on any given day. As dieters, we play the "I don't have time for exercise game." However, when you commit to 10,000 steps per day, you make walking a part of your lifestyle.

These feet were made for walking

As exercise, walking will restore your peace of mind, increase your mood and energy, help regulate your blood pressure and restore normal bodily functions. Walking is God-designed and is better than any pill or program invented by man. The human body is designed for walking. No one needs to be taught how to do it. However, we are walking for maximum impact and enjoyment. To start incorporating weekly walking as a part of your weight loss and wellness strategy and to get closer to your goal of *10,000* steps per day, see the following tips to get started:

1. Walk at least *30* minutes everyday.
2. Change your routes so that you are not walking on flat ground. If you live near hills or a beach, try different surface areas and elevations.
3. If you find it difficult to maintain a consistent brisk pace, you can alternate between a 4 minute brisk walk with a more comfortable pace for the next 4 minutes. After that 4 minute "rest", pick up your pace again.
4. If you can maintain brisk walk, do it for approximately *20* minutes.

Walking for, and on Purpose

You will not *accidentally* achieve 10,000 steps per day. I have counted my steps on days where I was at home for most of the day and I took as few as 700 steps! This new lifestyle will be gained by increasing steps in our normal, day to day activities, such as getting up to get the book across the room instead of asking your children to do it or walking to your co-workers area instead of e-mailing them. It is also setting aside time in the day for you, God and your body.

A better body through motion

When you feel your body in motion, you tap into the beauty of how God designed your body to move. You will build a healthy, strong and confident sense of self and well-being, along with increased strength. God desires for us to move and be a people of action and progressive motion. Let us not neglect this temple through inactivity, but let us move each day closer to the prize that lies before all of us. It is the sweetness of self-mastery, discipline and total surrender to God that pays the ultimate blessing and reward to us...a new body and a new life!

CHAPTER SEVEN

Seeking God's Hand and Not My Own

Operating in addictive patterns is oftentimes rooted in the spiritual issue of a lack of trust in God. We want the instant gratification that we supply ourselves through food. We fear the disappointment of waiting on God because somewhere in the back of our minds, we're afraid to be hurt or disappointed again.

Many overeaters substitute the discipline of waiting on God for the quick fix of our addictions. We shortchange ourselves by not feasting on what our soul truly longs for such as love, peace, forgiveness and acceptance. I believe that what God is holding in His hands for us, in a spiritual sense, is a whole lot better than anything we can get our hands on in the natural. When we reach a place of faith and obedience, where we can release the control and fully surrender, we will see the manifestation of what God has in store for us.

Matthew 7:7-11 "Ask, and it will be given to you; seek, and you will find; knock, and it will be opened to you. For everyone who asks receives, and he who seeks finds, and to him who knocks it will be opened. Or what man is there among you who, if his son asks for bread, will give him a stone? Or if he asks for a fish, will he give him a serpent? If you then, being evil, know how to give good gifts to your children, how much more will your Father who is in heaven give good things to those who ask Him!

Who is the provider in my life?

When people look at our lives as believers, they should see the provision of the Holy Spirit and not what we have provided ourselves through our momentary escapes with food that end up producing a physical and mental prison. When we are overweight and sick, bound to alcohol, stuck in unhealthy relationships and/or committed to beliefs in this world that have caused us to live below the greatness that God has intended for us, then you see *our* provision at work, not God's.

Do not seek success, seek God and success becomes inevitable

The more we focus on self means the more we focus on the things that we want in this world, the quick fix and the temporary things. The more we put our focus on the material success of this earth then the more we experience pain, anxiety, worry, doubt, fear, temptation and the struggle that this world brings. I'm not saying that we shouldn't want the best. I'm not saying that we shouldn't strive for an incredible life and live in excellence and work in excellence and achieve in excellence. However, we find greater peace and results when have to seek the provision, direction, wisdom and timing in His hand, not our own. Our success becomes a by-product of trusting in God.

You live in a small world when your world revolves around self

We must take our minds off a constant focus on our pain and inadequacies and place them on Christ.

Colossians 3:1-4 If then you were raised with Christ, seek those things which are above, where Christ is, sitting at the right hand of God. Set your mind on things above, not on things on the earth. For you died, and your life is hidden with Christ in God. When

Christ *who is* our life appears, then you also will appear with Him in glory.

Where our mind is, that's where our treasure is.

The enemy gains ground in this battle every time he gets our eyes off of God. It doesn't matter how he does it. It could be through a relationship. It could be through our doubt. It could be through our worry. It could be through our addictions. It could be through our struggles with our health. When we make focus on the reality of our struggle more than the healing power of God's Word, we set ourselves up for defeat.

On earth as it is in Heaven

Jesus taught the disciples to pray, "Your kingdom come. Your will be done on earth as *it is* in heaven" (Matthew 6:10). In Heaven, I have my new body, my victory, my provision. God's word says that the Kingdom of Heaven can be here on earth if I focus on the Kingdom of Heaven, and not solely on what my eyes see. Circumstance and current situations are subject to change. It does not take faith to speak what I see. The Bible says, "Now faith is the substance of things hoped for, the evidence of things not seen" (Hebrews 11:1).

Faith does not match logic, faith defies logic

It's not the size of the mountains we face, but the size of the God who promised to give us the mountain! If we take our eyes off of our limitations and fix our eyes on Jesus, He will lead us through to victory! Some friends and I were just speaking about how expensive the prices of homes are here in Southern California. It seems almost impossible for a family to purchase their first house here. However, the housing market does not move God. He operates by a different economic status. The Bible says that "the earth *is* the Lord's, and all its fullness" (Psalm 24:1).

Diets don't work...but Jesus does!

The bigger God becomes, the smaller my problems appear

If we can take the focus off of self and put it on God, He will become bigger and we'll become smaller. The more we increase God in our lives, the smaller we'll become. When we get to that place where we're fully trusting in God, we will witness breakthrough and provision. We can experience a present reality that mirrors our words, thoughts and deepest desires in Christ. If God gave you the vision, then He will give the provision.

God always provides for the vision He gives to us

God has given you a vision for a new body and life, for health and abundance. If God has given the vision, then He can provide everything necessary. He provides the power and authority through His Word and by the blood of Christ. By way of the Holy Spirit, He gives wisdom to instruct us in our care of His body temple.

One of the most powerful stories of trust and supernatural provision in the Bible is in Genesis. It is the story of Abraham and Sarah.

Genesis 22:1-18 Now it came to pass after these things that God tested Abraham, and said to him, "Abraham!" And he said, "Here I am." Then He said, "Take now your son, your only *son* Isaac, whom you love, and go to the land of Moriah, and offer him there as a burnt offering on one of the mountains of which I shall tell you." So Abraham rose early in the morning and saddled his donkey, and took two of his young men with him, and Isaac his son; and he split the wood for the burnt offering, and arose and went to the place of which God had told him. Then on the third day Abraham lifted his eyes and saw the place afar off. And Abraham said to his young men, "Stay here with the donkey; the lad and I will go yonder and worship, and we will come back to you." So Abraham took the wood of the burnt offering and laid *it* on Isaac his son; and he took the fire in his hand, and a knife, and the two of them went together. But Isaac spoke to Abraham his father and said, "My father!" And he said, "Here I am, my son." Then he said, "Look, the fire and the wood, but where *is* the lamb for a burnt offering?" And Abraham said, "My son, God will provide for Himself the lamb for a burnt offering." So the two of them went together. Then they came to the place of which God had told him. And Abraham built an altar there and placed the wood in order; and he bound Isaac his son and laid him on the altar, upon the wood. And Abraham stretched out his hand and took the knife to slay his son. But the Angel of the LORD called to him from heaven and said, "Abraham, Abraham!" So he said, "Here I am." And He said, "Do not lay your hand on the lad, or do anything to him; for now I know that you fear God, since you have not withheld your son, your only *son,* from Me."

Then Abraham lifted his eyes and looked, and there behind *him was* a ram caught in a thicket by its horns. So Abraham went and took the ram, and offered it up for a burnt offering instead of his son. And Abraham called the name of the place, The-LORD-Will-Provide; as it is said *to* this day, "In the Mount of the LORD it shall be provided." Then the Angel of the LORD called to Abraham a second time out of heaven, and said: "By Myself I have sworn, says the LORD, because you have done this thing, and have not withheld your son, your only *son—* blessing I will bless you, and multiplying I will multiply your descendants as the stars of the heaven and as the sand which *is* on the seashore; and your descendants shall possess the gate of their enemies. In your seed all the nations of the earth shall be blessed, because you have obeyed My voice."

What are you willing to surrender to God?

This story is so incredibly awesome. There can be no consistent victory without consistent sacrifice. A lot of us have made idols out of our fear and food. We have some things that we hold on to so tightly that we will not release them to God. Now here's Abraham, a man who was willing to offer his only son, whom he loved and was close to his heart. Abraham was available for God.

No sacrifice, no victory!

Some people are not willing to give up a meal for God, let alone a piece of candy. The temporary pleasure this world offers can become idols in our heart. We are not willing to give our careers, ambitions and/or desires to God because we're afraid if we give them to Him that He will not give them back to us. Abraham was prepared for the journey, knowing that God was a God of power and promise. This is not a weight problem this is a heart problem. Our obesity is the result of exalting food and eating in our hearts. It is time to sacrifice our temporary self-pleasure for lasting promise.

Waiting on God as it relates to hunger

Waiting on God's timing and provision go hand in hand with the natural principle of waiting on true hunger. True hunger is a vulnerable place. Most overweight dieter's associate pain with being hungry, so we eat before our bodies ever call for food. Yet when I wait on God's natural timing for my body, not only will I enjoy the food that much more, but I can relish in the freedom of waiting. Waiting requires trust, love and faith. Are you willing to wait on God? Our body is the place of reverence and honor. Everyday, we are given the opportunity to worship through our obedience.

Experiencing the provision of God daily

When we sacrifice on a daily basis and we show God that we want what He has more than what we have, then we will see the majesty, glory and provision of the Lord operating in our lives. In such a place, we will stand in awe daily of how our God is a God who provides for, takes care of and loves his people.

CHAPTER EIGHT

Living in the Moment

Over my years of counseling and ministering to thousands of men and women, of teaching in different and various workshops and working with various congregations, I've realized that many of us are the *walking wounded.* We hang on to words that were spoken into our lives, the abuses suffered, the disappointments and the hurts. We are still holding on to them because we can not properly express the pain. We can't share and put our minds around what it is that we feel and the *religious mentality* has wounded and prevented so many of us from truly having a consistent relationship with God. So, we stuff the pain with food and silence our heart's cry.

Seeing God in the moment

God is found in the moment. God is calling us to live in the now, because God is a very present help in trouble. He can heal you now from your past. However, God is no longer in your past and neither are you. All throughout the Word God calls people of faith to move out of their zone of comfort and He challenges them in that new place to be strong, have faith and go to a different level of believing in Him!

Living in the moment is taking responsibility and action

Obesity was caused by allowing ourselves to "go unconscious", becoming inactive and numbing ourselves with food. To walk in victory requires conscious presence and awareness of our actions, thoughts and habits which will propel us into a new moment of triumph. Living in the moment is taking responsibility and ownership over our choices.

Joshua 1:1-9 After the death of Moses the servant of the LORD, it came to pass that the LORD spoke to Joshua the son of Nun, Moses' assistant, saying: "Moses My servant is dead. Now therefore, arise, go over this Jordan, you and all this people, to the land which I am giving to them—the children of Israel. Every place that the sole of your foot will tread upon I have given you, as I said to Moses. From the wilderness and this Lebanon as far as the great river, the River Euphrates, all the land of the Hittites, and to the Great Sea toward the going down of the sun, shall be your territory. No man shall *be able to* stand before you all the days of your life; as I was with Moses, *so* I will be with you. I will not leave you nor forsake you. Be strong and of good courage, for to this people you shall divide as an inheritance the land which I swore to their fathers to give them. Only be strong and very courageous, that you may observe to do according to all the law which Moses My servant commanded you; do not turn from it to the right hand or to the left, that you may prosper wherever you go. This Book of the Law shall not depart from your mouth, but you shall meditate in it day and night, that you may observe to do according to all that is written in it. For then you will make your way prosperous, and then you will have good success. Have I not commanded you? Be strong and of good courage; do not be afraid, nor be dismayed, for the LORD your God *is* with you wherever you go."

God is calling us into a new life

Looking at the life of Joshua, we see that this was a man who was brought up under Moses' great leadership. Joshua, at the time of Moses' death, had to assume a position of leadership for the people of that nation. It was a lot of pressure to fall upon Joshua's shoulders. In times of pressure and new responsibilities, we are tempted to shrink back in fear. Joshua could have easily dwelt in the past. He could have focused on how things could, should or would be if Moses were still alive. Instead, he rose to the challenge. Joshua answered God's call to be courageous as he laid claim on the promise of new land and blessings.

Rise to the challenge of living in the moment

When we make a decision to leave our past of overeating and shame and move into the place of now, God challenges us to be strong and courageous knowing that He's with us *always*. God's challenge to Joshua is followed by a promise to him. God can make it so that everywhere you step, you have dominion and authority over your enemies. He says to Joshua, "Be strong and of good courage." I love when he tells Joshua to be strong, because being strong is something that we have to do in the moment. It takes courage to walk in the moment of God's favor and direction.

Great purpose in pain

I know in the past that we have been through some dark places and have not felt that God was with us. We have not felt God's protection because of the pain or abuse we have suffered at the hands of others. We ask God, "Why would you allow this to happen to me?" "Why would you allow this to happen to my child or my family?" With all of my dark days and moments of anguish, I have learned that there is great purpose in pain. It is a tool that can focus us and cause us to let go of distraction and prioritize our spiritual life. It can make us bitter or better. Pain is a tool that can shape a life by the power that we give it, and the choices we make in spite of it. This is why you can have two people with similar stories of abuse. One person goes on to use their pain for purpose, pours into the lives of others and is refreshed by the building and loving of other hurt souls. The other person is stuck and blinded by the pain and cannot separate what has happened to them from who they truly are. They become bitter and never see the fullness of God's Word when He promises that "all things work together for good to those who love God, to those who are called according to His purpose" (Romans 8:28).

The blessing in the trial

I have reached a point in my walk where I am so grateful for all of my trials. I am learning to stop begging God to "deliver" me out of the trial into my blessing. It is a sweet place to realize that the blessing is found within the trial. In the hard times, God is shaping me, molding me, healing my deepest pain and transforming into His likeness through the fellowship of suffering. I know this does not line up with modern day "feel good" preaching, but it is Biblical to see God in every season of life, and to learn the freedom of gratitude no matter what the outer circumstance is.

James 1:2-4 My brethren, count it all joy when you fall into various trials, knowing that the testing of your faith produces patience. But let patience have *its* perfect work, that you may be perfect and complete, lacking nothing.

My experience does not outweigh God's word

The Bible says "many are the afflictions of the righteous, but the Lord delivers him out of them all" (Psalm 34:19). We have the power to choose not to allow our personal life experiences to negate or outweigh God's Word. We limit God's authority to influence our lives when we limit His Word.

My outlook determines my view and experience in life.

When God says that He will supply all of my needs according to His riches and glory (Philippians 4:19), does it matter that my bank account is in the negative? When God says that He will heal all of my diseases (Psalm 103:3), does it matter that I have cancer? Does it matter that I have heart disease or Lupus? Does it matter that I'm still struggling with an illness? When God says that I am more than a conqueror (Romans 8:37), does it matter that I struggle momentarily with overeating? Faith does not confess and speak on the current circumstance. True faith makes you a master of the circumstance, not a servant to it. When I walk by faith, I choose to believe God's Word and accept it in the moment. Before I ever *see* my change, belief must take firm root in my heart. Belief in my heart creates actions that reflect my beliefs. God says to meditate on His Word (Joshua 1:8). to be strong and be of good courage because it takes strength and courage to live in the now.

Are you living life for the joy of the moment?

Wake up and smell the roses, play with your kids, look out at nature without worrying about the future or dwelling in the past. There's a joy that comes when you can sit with your spouse and have a healthy conversation, not dwelling on everything that you didn't do two years ago or everything that you didn't say two weeks ago. Instead, you can be present, right here and now. There's a wonderful joy that comes from being in the moment.

Dwelling in the past paralyzes us from moving in the moment

2 Timothy 1:7 For God has not given us a spirit of fear, but of power and of love and of a sound mind.

Jesus is the author and finisher of our faith. When our decisions are based on the disappointments of our past, we are not led by wisdom or the mind of Christ.

Philippians 3:13-14 Brethren, I do not count myself to have apprehended; but one thing *I do,* forgetting those things which are behind and reaching forward to those things which are ahead, I press toward the goal for the prize of the upward call of God in Christ Jesus.

When we dwell in the past, we may miss the leading of God to make proper decisions in the moment. We have a tendency to make choices from a place of fear, loss, rejection or hurt. When we renounce our past and accept our newness in Christ, we are liberated from guilt and shame!

2 Corinthians 5:17 Therefore, if anyone *is* in Christ, *he is* a new creation; old things have passed away; behold, all things have become new.

A new creation lives in the moment

When we give our lives, our past, our shame and our hurt to Jesus, it becomes hidden in Christ. Everyday we need the cleansing blood of Christ to wash us clean from all the things that we may be holding onto from our past. A new creation in Christ lives for the joy, revelation and victory of the moment.

How does living in the moment affect our eating?

We overeat when we're in a place of looking at past hurts. We punish ourselves with food. We stuff the pain. When our past brings up feelings of unworthiness, self-hatred or doubt, we further that abuse cycle when we reach for food. We use food to *eat at people*, to get back at those who have hurt us. The past will keep us bound in a cycle of failure until we allow ourselves the freedom of life in the moment.

Psalm 46:1-2 God *is* our refuge and strength, A very present help in trouble. Therefore we will not fear, Even though the earth be removed, and though the mountains be carried into the midst of the sea.

God is a very present help.

What is it that you need help with now? What past hurt are you willing to release in order to experience lasting freedom? When we cast our cares on God and accept the challenge of letting go of our past, we will experience the breakthrough, the provision and the blessing of the moment. One moment in the presence of God can transform our entire lives. We must never underestimate the transforming power of a moment in God's presence. Give God your *inner weights* of shame, guilt, fear and doubt. Allow His transforming and healing power to operate through you, as you shed the *outer weight*. God does not need you to "work for Him" He desires to work *through* you, in *this* very moment. Will you yield your very soul to His touch? When you live a life of surrender each moment with Jesus is sweeter than the one before!

CHAPTER NINE

Self-Love for Weight Loss Success

What's love got to do with it?

What does a person who loves herself look like? What does she act like? What does her lifestyle reflect? What is her passion? When we love ourselves, it should reflect in every single thing we do. Self-love is a huge part of weight loss success. Overweight dieters often say, "When I get sick and tired and disgusted enough with myself, I'll make changes." "I hate my thighs. I hate my hips. I hate my legs. I hate my arms, I hate the way my body looks. I hate the way my face looks. I hate the kinds of decisions that I make." These negative thoughts and self-deprecating beliefs that we hold do not motivate us to lasting change. Instead, they encourage the cycle of overeating, shame and guilt.

Jesus, do you think I'm pretty?

Genesis 1:26 Then God said, "Let Us make man in Our image, according to Our likeness; let them have dominion over the fish of the sea, over the birds of the air, and over the cattle, over all the earth and over every creeping thing that creeps on the earth." Wonderful. Powerful. Wise. Magnificent. Beautiful. Lovely. Incredible. Glorious. These are words that do not even begin to scratch the surface when we describe the awesomeness of God. Yet God says, "let us make man in our image, in our own likeness." When you look up the word likeness, it means reflection. We are to reflect God's image, beauty, love and grace.

The world's view of beauty

We live in a world that bombards us with thousands of ad campaigns per day that send a subtle message that we are not enough. We are not thin enough, smart enough, famous enough, pretty enough or rich enough. So, when we spend our efforts trying to become a reflection of the world instead of reflecting God, we end up with poor self-esteem, low confidence, insecurities and a genuine lack of self-love and respect.

Seeing myself through God's eyes

God does not want our standards of acceptance, love or beauty to be based on the world's view. True esteem, beauty and confidence come from knowing who we are and whose we are. The Bible says that I was formed in God's image. Yet, when I look at my life, my body and my reality, they may not outwardly reflect the marvelous splendor of God. In 2 Corinthians 3:18, the Word promises that God is moving me from "glory to glory" and when I recognize my beauty and magnificence comes from the hands of a divine Master craftsman, I can yield myself to His molding, His shaping and His desires for my life. Then, I will truly see the fruition of His promises to make my life His poem.

Ephesians 2:10 For we are His workmanship, created in Christ Jesus for good works, which God prepared beforehand that we should walk in them.

I am God's poetry

When God calls me His *workmanship,* it simply means I am His *poem,* His work of art. My life should tell the story of His goodness, grace and love. Currently, there are DVDs that allow the viewer to select the ending of the movie by choosing between alternate endings. In real life, we also have a hand in telling our own life's story. We can chose to accept the truth that we are God's most beautiful and wonderful work. I am a nature buff, partly because it keeps me in awe of God's unlimited power and extraordinary creativity. When I peer into a sky that is painted with shades of pink, purple and brilliant hues of blue, I say, "Wow! God is beautiful." And yet, I know that I am more beautiful than anything in this creation because out of all of God's most magnificent works of art in nature, He says that *I* am made in His image. I reflect Him. He did not say that about the beautiful oceans, the white sand beaches, the snow-capped mountain peaks, nor the splendor of the eagle as it takes flight. But for me, He poured in His utmost greatness. How dare I see myself as anything less; how dare I insult a Holy God by not honoring, loving and respecting *His* most marvelous creation…*me*.

Self-love is a part of the journey towards wholeness.

Loving ourselves is a healing practice and will produce powerful results. We must forget what our mothers or fathers did or did not say and allow ourselves to find love in the arms of a Heavenly Father who looks down upon us and smiles at the splendor of His creation. The gift that God gives to us is one of choice. And how I treat others is a direct reflection of choosing to remember God's love for me and giving that love freely to others. When Jesus died on the cross, He paid the ultimate sacrifice. I believe that He paid for the sins of self-contempt, self-hatred and self-loathing. Many of us find it incredibly easy to say, "I'm just hard on myself," "Well, I'm just critical of myself," "I just want to make sure I take inventory of my faults." However, when this kind of self-introspection reaches a place of being damaging and affecting us on a subconscious level, we are sabotaging ourselves and short-changing our potential in Christ. Our low self-esteem has become a hindrance to purpose and discovering our greatness through God's word.

Ephesians 5:28-29 So husbands ought to love their own wives as their own bodies; he who loves his wife loves himself. For no one ever hated his own flesh, but nourishes and cherishes it, just as the Lord *does* the church.

Are you a self-hater?

The Bible says that no one has ever hated their own flesh. If the husband loves the wife, he should love the wife as he loves his own body, and vice versa. I want to love my husband as I love myself. I want to love my neighbor as I love myself, but how can I if I'm in a cycle of self-hatred or self-loathing? When I look out at this world and I focus on what society tells me I *should* be, what I *should* look like, what I *should* have attained by now, I can fall into a cycle of self-contempt.

Love our neighbor as we love ourselves

The Word charges the husband to love his wife as he loves his own body. What do you do when you're married to a man who does not love himself? Will that affect you? Absolutely! As women, what about when we say, "I love my husband, but I have a hard time with me?" Unfortunately, the hard time that we have with ourselves is eventually going to manifest itself in our relationship. How I treat myself is only a reflection of how I will eventually treat others. I remember the changes that occurred in my body after I had my first two sons. I began to examine myself constantly in an unhealthy way. I became disgusted with my less than perky breasts, my excess weight and my loose, saggy skin. I became so focused on how uncomfortable I was that I missed the moments for God to build me up in quiet times of prayer. I avoided His affirmation almost like it was a mirror. It became familiar and comforting to be hard on myself. When I was looking at self, my eyes were not on Jesus.

Isaiah 26:3 You will keep *him* in perfect peace, *Whose* mind *is* stayed *on You,* Because he trusts in You.

Being overly self-conscious robs us of our peace

I was not living in peace. I was conscious of my body and it affected my relationship and communication with my husband. I couldn't understand why he didn't support my self critiques and co-sign on my desires for plastic surgery and radical change. I missed the fact that God still loved me through my husband's patience and desire. I did not see myself through God's eyes. Instead, I saw myself in the limitations of the mirror. I needed to be healed first in my heart so that my body would follow.

Physical beauty is limited

By the world's standards, I am a fairly smart and attractive woman. Yet, how I feel about my beauty comes from the inside because there will always be someone prettier, smarter and more successful than I am. Women who base their self-esteem on looks are bound in the prison of comparison and self-examination. It is liberating to realize that physical beauty has its limitations but in Christ I have a unique purpose, destiny and gifts. I truly have an inner beauty that this world can never shake nor take away from me.

Proverbs 31:30 Charm *is* deceitful and beauty *is* passing, But a woman *who* fears the LORD, she shall be praised.

Can physical beauty satisfy us?

I have friends who are successful Hollywood actresses who are gorgeous and indeed could set beauty standards and trends in their own right. However, I have never met a satisfied woman who was not connected to her Maker. Most women will find fault or issue with something about their bodies or appearance. The enemy is a liar and he always perverts natural desires. As women, we desire to look our best and be our best. I believe God wired us that way. However, when our outward appearance becomes all-consuming, and reaches a place of vanity, or on the opposite end, extreme self-consciousness, doubt and comparison, we have fallen into the world's destructive system of obsessive self driven thoughts.

How does a lack of self-love affect the overeater?

When I'm *constantly* thinking about myself, thinking about what's wrong with me, about the mistakes I've made, how I don't measure up, how I don't fit in, thinking how I'm not as educated, as gifted, as beautiful, as wealthy, all the things that I'm not - what kind of emotions does these bring up? These thoughts are accompanied by feelings of unworthiness, shame, doubt and depression. As emotional eaters, these feelings further the cycle of overeating. It is my desire to see the body of Christ, especially women in the body of Christ, rise up from the ashes of defeat in our past and our own mind, and recognize our individual purpose, beauty, strength and value.

It is okay for me to love myself

Because when I love myself, it's easier for me to love my neighbor. When I love myself, I am in agreement with God's Word and when I agree with God's Word, I align myself with the creative power of God's most abundant blessings to overflow in my life.

Eating like I love myself

We have detailed in this book the natural eating principles necessary for lasting weight loss success:

One: Waiting on and responding to True Physical Hunger. Eating only when you are truly physically hungry. Not from mental hunger, not from emotional hunger, not from spiritual hunger, but from true physical (stomach) hunger.

Two: Eating to the point of comfortable satisfaction. We will not gorge or stuff ourselves to the point of pain, discomfort, self-abuse or gluttony.

Three: Wise Eating. Using and exercising wisdom in my personal eating choices. Taking responsibility over my own health and food choices and eating the foods that are agreeable and favorable to my body.

Practicing love at each meal

We are more important than the next bite of food. We are worthy of experiencing freedom and victory. When we eat from a standpoint of grace, self-nurturing and love at each and every meal, we can choose to end the cycle of overeating, self-abuse, guilt and doubt. Each new day will offer us the opportunity to eat or to not eat from a standpoint of love. It takes great strength to love others. It takes even greater strength to love ourselves. Our eating habits will be a direct reflection of how much we love and care for our own personal well-being.

Loving myself takes time....

If we don't take time to nourish and feed ourselves, then how can we be expected to feed other people? We give our time and our attention to the things that we value. If you are not aggressive and adamant about taking care of yourself, it may affect the degree of kindness and generosity that you can give to your children, family and your peers - emotionally, physically and spiritually. Taking moments to take care of ourselves is crucial for weight loss and wellness.

Loving myself requires trust

It is time to rise to the purpose to which God has called us. When God created me, He created something wonderful and extraordinary. God said that He made me in His own image, so hating myself is hating the creation of God. Doubting myself, in essence, doubts God. Not trusting the gifts, talents and abilities that God put in me does, in essence, not trust the Creator. When I look at myself and try to fashion myself after this world, I fail to utilize and capitalize on the uniqueness that God has placed in my life and personality. Our quirkiness, our little idiosyncrasies help fashion us into God's purpose.

God is not a cookie-cutter God

If you start to resemble the world or another person or group of people, be afraid, be very afraid because you may be on the path to losing *you*. We find ourselves in the pages of life, outlined in God's Word. We find ourselves again in the simple quiet moments of honesty and attention to our own soul. Nobody can be who God has called you to be, you are rare and unique. Self-love is very powerful. It should look very powerful. Loving myself will begin to translate into how I treat my physical body. The time, care and nurturing attention that I invest in myself will yield high spiritual and natural returns.

Loving myself takes forgiveness

One of the greatest ways I love myself is to forgive others. Unforgiveness keeps me bound, eating or is self-abuse. I am yielding the power of my thought-life, actions and feelings to someone else's control. Forgiveness is much more for me than it is the other person. It is setting them free from what I feel they owe me and giving myself the ability to walk in a new life unencumbered by the pain to which unforgiveness binds me. Part of my process of loving myself is realizing that just because people in my past have hurt me or disappointed me does not mean I am not worthy of freedom and goodness.

True liberty is being free from people

When I keep myself in a position of purpose, moving forward and seeking God's best for my life, then my outlook and view changes for the better. I, like Joseph, can reach a place of understanding and believe that what was meant for evil, God used it for good. In Genesis 37, we learn that Joseph was sold into slavery by his own brothers who then lied to his father and told him that Joseph was dead. He was imprisoned, falsely accused and lost his mother, who died during the time that he was separated from his family. Joseph knew what prison in the natural felt like. I believe that he loved himself and the plan of God enough to not subject himself to prison again - the prison of unforgiveness. So, if you are holding on to an offense, go to your brother like the Bible instructs or let it go and trust God to heal your heart and restore or correct the situation. Whichever you do, love yourself enough to get free from people in your past. Those constant "re-plays" in your mind only keep you in a place of defeat and self sabotage. It's time to walk in love with your Maker and yourself. Love brings freedom and liberty, and true liberty is being free from people! Free to change. Free to love God with a clean heart.

Where does confidence or lack of confidence begin?

Philippians 3:3 For we are the circumcision, who worship God in the Spirit, rejoice in Christ Jesus, and have no confidence in the flesh.

My lack of confidence comes from looking at my flesh. Likewise, many other people base their confidence in the flesh and the things in the natural are ever changing. However, God says I can have a form of confidence, power and faith that has nothing to do with situation, circumstance or flesh.

Philippians 3:4-7 though I also might have confidence in the flesh. If anyone else thinks he may have confidence in the flesh, I more so: circumcised the eighth day, of the stock of Israel, *of* the tribe of Benjamin, a Hebrew of the Hebrews; concerning the law, a Pharisee; concerning zeal, persecuting the church; concerning the righteousness which is in the law, blameless. But what things were gain to me, these I have counted loss for Christ.

Paul, if you want to compare him to today's politicians, was the President. If you want to talk about money, he was the wealthiest person in the world. If you want to talk about beauty, he was the most handsome man on the face of the planet. And yet, when he found Christ, he had no confidence in any of those former things. His confidence was in the Lord.

Philippians 3:8 Yet indeed I also count all things loss for the excellence of the knowledge of Christ Jesus my Lord, for whom I have suffered the loss of all things, and count them as rubbish, that I may gain Christ.

Confidence found in purpose

So many of us are trying to gain things in the world to make ourselves *okay*. I always say the root of confidence is in knowing why you are here on earth. Find out what your purpose is and it won't matter if you're the best looking woman in the room. It won't matter if you have the newest pair of shoes. You will know that you are doing what the Creator has called on you to do. I am the richest woman in the room because I have the love of Christ. I have the knowledge of Christ. I have the salvation and acceptance of the Lord Jesus Christ. I have what so many other people are seeking; I have unconditional, unwavering love, and a clear unwavering vision of my purpose.

Love empowers you to change

Tapping into that truth gives me the tool to push away from the plate and to establish a healthy relationship with food. It allows me the freedom to be transformed in my mind, body and spirit by God's Word. This truth allows me to embrace my new body and life with passion, not bound by the sin of unworthiness. Receiving the truth that I am God's greatest miracle should manifest changes in my daily actions. It's awesome to know that of all the places on this wondrous planet He could choose to reside, He chose my body as a resting place for His Spirit. We have the power, wisdom, beauty, grace and favor of God's Holy Spirit dwelling within our bodies. Think about this… God sees you as His most precious creation, beautiful and magnificent. Why should you be the one to disagree?

CHAPTER TEN

How Faith Wins at Weight Loss

John 5:2-8 Now there is in Jerusalem by the Sheep *Gate* a pool, which is called in Hebrew, Bethesda, having five porches. In these lay a great multitude of sick people, blind, lame, paralyzed, waiting for the moving of the water. For an angel went down at a certain time into the pool and stirred up the water; then whoever stepped in first, after the stirring of the water, was made well of whatever disease he had. Now a certain man was there who had an infirmity thirty-eight years. When Jesus saw him lying there, and knew that he already had been *in that condition* a long time, He said to him, "Do you want to be made well?" The sick man answered Him, "Sir, I have no man to put me into the pool when the water is stirred up; but while I am coming, another steps down before me." Jesus said to him, "Rise, take up your bed and walk." And immediately the man was made well, took up his bed, and walked. And that day was the Sabbath.

Imagine five porches filled with the sick, outcast, lowly and destitute, who have traveled from all corners of the nations to reach this marvelous place. A place where an angel descends from Heaven to trouble the waters and healing is promised to anyone who reaches the water at that miraculous time. I have long been fascinated with this man, but more so with his journey to this place.

Have you ever been disappointed while waiting on God?

Who brought him to the healing waters of Bethesda 38 years ago? A mother, a father, a cousin? How long did they stay with him before he was abandoned and left to his own resources? Who sent him a message early in his life that he was not worthy of healing, being free? What caused him to believe that he was bound by his current circumstance and surrounding? I wondered how many days he looked upon the other ill people whose families stayed with them, supporting them in love. I wondered if at night he dreamed "this is it. Tomorrow, I am going to get in first," only to be wounded by his own faith, hurt by his own unfulfilled expectations of healing. How many nights did he struggle with loneliness feeling like God had forgotten him? How did he feel on this, his *38th* year having seen thousands come in sick and leave out healed, and yet he lay there seemingly worse off than when he was first brought to this place of promise?

The most important question we can ask ourselves

His entire life was about to change if he could answer one question correctly. On the day that Jesus entered that place, He had an eagle eye focus for this man. Jesus sought him out and did not lay hands upon him and heal him instantly like He had the power to do. Instead, He asked a simple yet profound question: *Do you want to be made well?*

It's time to speak your innermost desires

I wondered why Jesus would ask him that question when the answer seemed so obvious. Of course, he wanted to be better. Doesn't everyone? But, I do not think so. People can derive comfort from complaining. They can gain attention from their illness. Research has shown that AIDS patients actually become depressed when their sickness goes into remission. The disease begins to define them and when they are no longer sick, it's time to face the real world again and that can be frightening. I believe Jesus asked him this question because He wanted the man with his own mouth to speak hope back into his life. When the man offered excuses for his condition, Jesus saw the *yes* in his heart, the yes he was afraid to say. Like many of us, he was wounded by the pain of disappointment.

Are you ready to abandon your excuses to gain freedom?

We become afraid to ask for what our heart truly desires. But, Jesus saw the heart and Jesus can take our hope, inspire us to faith and then direct us into action. Jesus reminded him of why he began his journey 38 years ago. It was not to sit on the outside of the blessing looking in, but to experience it for himself. All the reasons and excuses disappeared. He did not need the excuse of no one helping him to the water, for he was in the presence of Jesus…the living water. When he said yes, he was saying, "I am now ready to leave the comfort of my painful surroundings and to venture out into the life You have for me."

Faith and action are one

Jesus commanded him to pick up his bed and walk. I believe that we all have a "bed" in our lives, and when we say yes to Jesus, he causes us to rise up and leave the bed behind. The bed is symbolic of our fear, our dependence on the flesh and our dependence on the thoughts of this world. When we lie down on a bed of self-reliance, we may look like we are getting closer to the promise, closer to the breakthrough, but the reality of the circumstance keeps us bound in disappointment and frustration. The *world* says, "God helps those who help themselves." The Word of God says the opposite. Scripture tells us that God helps and directs those who are humble enough to admit they cannot do it in their own strength (Psalm 25:9).

Do you want to be made well?

Then we must realize the role that faith plays in our wellness and weight loss. Faith is hope, belief and action. Faith is not based on what we see with our eyes, but what we are trusting for in our hearts. So, before we ever see the manifestation in the natural of our new body, we must first see and accept the truth of God's promise of healing and restoration in our hearts.

In Christ the rules for our success have changed

When we come to Christ, we transfer into a different kingdom. The kingdom of the world says, "I'll believe it when I see it." In contrast, the Kingdom of God is different because the Word of God says to focus on the things that are unseen. Focus on the Kingdom and all other things will be added unto you (Matthew 6:33). Don't seek after what you're going to eat, drink or wear, but focus on a God that is not seen and all the things that you need will be given to you in the natural. It's a completely different Kingdom. Our visions and dreams of a new body, life, ministry and purpose are already a reality when we see it through the eyes of faith.

2 Corinthians 5:17 Therefore, if anyone *is* in Christ, *he is* a new creation; old things have passed away; behold, all things have become new.

Faith is the substance of things hoped for, the evidence of things not seen (Hebrew 11:1). I have evidence when I look at my bank account that I am not rich. However, I know what I hope for and I stand by faith on the provision that God has promised me in His Word. I have evidence or facts when I look in the mirror that my body is not the way I might desire for it to look, but I have faith in what I hope for when I say, "God, I know that I'm a new creation. I know that my body is transformed, that my health is transformed." Faith has nothing to do with the facts. It has absolutely nothing to do with supporting evidence, it is the exact opposite. I live by faith when I believe for what I cannot see in the natural. I train myself to see the promises of God within my heart first.

Galatians 3:11 But that no one is justified by the law in the sight of God *is* evident, for *"the just shall live by faith."*

Faith and logic will forever be in direct opposition with one another, clashing with one another. God sees my life from beginning to end. Our view is limited. When I come to God, I must believe that He *is* and I must also believe that He is a rewarder of those who diligently seek Him (Hebrews 11:6). I seek out God by faith, not by sight. I say, "God, I come to church every Sunday. I worship You. I sing songs of praise to a God that I've never seen. When I go to bed at night, I pray to a God that I've never met. But I know that by Your Spirit, by the promises in Your Word, by the revelation of Your anointing and Your will, and by Your power and presence in my life, You're real." I know that I walk by faith and not by sight. So, if I live my life serving a God that I can't see, I also want to live my life by the promises of God's Word which I can see. I want to take Him completely at His Word.

Habakkuk 2:2-3 Then the LORD answered me and said: "Write the vision and make *it* plain on tablets, that he may run who reads it. For the vision *is* yet for an appointed time; but at the end it will speak, and it will not lie. Though it tarries, wait for it; because it will surely come, it will not tarry.

The vision that God has for our lives is for an appointed time. Even if I don't see my new body or life yet, it is still finished. We must align our actions and daily steps with God's promises. Because we will act on what we believe and pretty soon we manifest it in our lives.

The just shall speak by faith…

Proverbs 18:21 Death and life *are* in the power of the tongue, And those who love it will eat its fruit.

The Bible says that there is life and death in the power of the tongue and so many of us have been speaking death over ourselves instead of life. We have been speaking death over our bodies instead of life. What have you been speaking by faith into your own life? What have you been speaking into the lives of those around you?

We can use our tongue to betray and hurt or we can use our tongue to build up, edify and encourage.

Matthew 24:35 Heaven and earth will pass away, but My words will by no means pass away.

God gave the tool of speech and communication to us as one of the most powerful weapons in the world. I personally believe my voice is one of the most powerful tools I have. By mere words, wars have begun. By words, wars have ceased. God spoke the world into existence. His Word is full of power and life. It will not change or pass away. So when we utilize His Word, by faith, as an instrument in our own lives, our lives begin to take on a different shape and so do our physical bodies. Whatever we fail to conquer will eventually conquer us. Begin speaking words of victory and allow your *walk* to model your *talk*.

Have you ever been called fat? Have you ever been called ugly?

We invest faith in the lies that others have spoken over us when we live out their words and demonstrate that behavior in our daily actions. When we live our lives by the Word of God and not by words that other people have spoken over us, we will see victory, healing, weight loss and change. When we are meditating or rehashing their words of negativity over and over again and our meditation of the heart becomes our action. That is why we must meditate on the Word of God, so our actions model His word.

Psalm 119:9-16 How can a young man cleanse his way? By taking heed according to Your word. With my whole heart I have sought You; Oh, let me not wander from Your commandments! Your word I have hidden in my heart, That I might not sin against You. Blessed *are* You, O LORD! Teach me Your statutes. With my lips I have declared All the judgments of Your mouth. I have rejoiced in the way of Your testimonies, As *much as* in all riches. I will meditate on Your precepts, And contemplate Your ways. I will delight myself in Your statutes; I will not forget Your word.

Words can shape our bodies and lives

Many of us used to sing that song, "sticks and stones may break my bones, but names will never hurt me." Nothing could be further from the truth because if we allow them to, the words that have been spoken to us can yield a creative kind of power to shape our lives. God wants me to meditate, seek and remind myself constantly of His Word. When I come to a place where I say, Lord, I am trusting You for renewed health, I'm trusting You for a new body and life and yet my words speak the exact opposite, I am shaping my reality by the words that I speak. If I get up everyday and say, - "Lord, I present my body as a living sacrifice, holy and acceptable to You. I know that my body is not my own. You have fearfully and wonderfully made me. My body is Your temple and I will govern myself accordingly by my words." - then I will create a new reality in my life.

People, who are hurting inside, hurt others with their words

Luke 6:45 A good man out of the good treasure of his heart brings forth good; and an evil man out of the evil treasure of his heart brings forth evil. For out of the abundance of the heart his mouth speaks.

I remember being pregnant and newly married. I was so insecure about the way my body looked that I would find myself saying little negative remarks about other women. I didn't feel good about myself, because I wasn't confident in the Lord. My lack of self-love translated into a harsh and critical nature with others and I knew that this was not God's design for my tongue. I knew that according to His design for my life, my words were to edify, build, create and speak life and love.

How does faith begin?

Faith is a belief in our hearts that should translate into solid, consistent action.

James 2:14 What does it profit, my brethren, if someone says he has faith but does not have works? Can faith save him?

Are Christians lazy and complacent?

Before I became a believer, I was ambitious and focused. I was the person who always had a business plan in hand and I diligently pursued success. When I was in the world, I would look at the church and Christians and I would say, "Christians seem lazy to me. They seem like they're always just sitting around, waiting on Jesus." Later, I realized I was looking at the *wrong* Christians. I realized that Christians who are walking by faith are in a consistent place of movement. They are stepping out on hope. They are stepping out on conviction. They are stepping out on persuasion. They are taking daily action to realize their dreams and vision, because faith without works is dead (James 2:14).

Faith should be accompanied by plans and actions

It's nothing for me to say that I know God has given me a vision of having a new home if I never call the broker's office; if I never step out on faith and start looking for homes and going to open houses. It means nothing for me to say that I believe God has given me a vision or an idea for a business. Yet, I never get my business cards, name, logo or license. A lot of us ride on that grace boat, sailing down a river of religious-based complacency and we're not in true faith because true faith looks like something. True faith is movement. True faith is conviction. It's a persuasion plus a corresponding action that directly affects my outcome.

My daily actions are a direct result of my faith/belief

I say, "God, I believe that I'm healed in the name of Jesus." What is my corresponding action to that? I'm going to speak God's Word. I'm going to stand on God's Word. I'm going to claim my healing and my deliverance. I'm also going to do whatever else in the natural that God has called me to do. My faith is still in God, but my actions are a direct result of my faith.

Applying your faith/action to weight loss

We say D*iets don't work...but Jesus does*. So, what is Jesus doing in your life? How is that manifesting itself in real, tangible, physical and spiritual change? What are we doing to step that promise of victory out in the natural? Are we diligently applying the natural eating principles outlined in this book that will usher in our weight loss success? When worldly diets come along and tell us to do A, B and C, we'll do it. We will submit ourselves to the diet laws of man because somewhere in our hearts we believe that we will see results. But when God says, "Push away from the plate when you're not hungry. Do not eat to excess. Do not seek food for comfort. Seek Me." What is my corresponding action to that?

Are you waiting for rain, or preparing before clouds to form?

Look at the Biblical faith hero Noah in Genesis 6. He built the ark long before the rain ever came because he was convicted in his heart. He had a persuasion in his heart that if God says it, then it is true. Success is when preparation and opportunity meet face to face. Are we prepared, are we ready? Many times, we're waiting on God to do something. "Well, I'm just waiting on God. I'm just waiting on God to do something." Meanwhile, God is saying, "You do the possible; let... me do the impossible!"

Losing weight by faith

I challenge you that when you're not physically hungry, *don't eat*. That's your faith. That's your corresponding action, push away from the plate, choose something different or delay gratification or start walking. My corresponding action is to get into prayer. My corresponding action is to take things into my body that are going to keep my system clean and healthy. My corresponding action is to say, "Lord, I'm putting you first before anything in this world."

My daily faith is to submit and surrender to God. As believers, our lives need to be about action, not complacency. We need to start trusting that God will lead us and guide us into lasting victory and as we move by faith we will experience first hand how faith wins at weight loss!

CHAPTER ELEVEN

Worship Over Weight

Could you be hungry for more of Jesus?

We overeat because we are empty. We stuff ourselves, yet are never satisfied. We get full, yet are never really filled because we confuse the signals of physical and spiritual hunger. Most of us are hungry for more of Jesus. We're really hungry for more of God. We are really hungry for more of His presence, His Word, His anointing and His direction. When we overcome our dependency on and idolatry of food, we can hear from God in a whole new and awe- inspiring way.

Matthew 4:4 But He answered and said, "It is written, *'Man shall not live by bread alone, but by every word that proceeds from the mouth of God.'"*

Jesus was not on a "spiritual low-carb" diet

Jesus knew that in order to have true life on earth, He must feast on the Word of God which the Bible says is the bread of life (Luke 4:4). Jesus is our portion. Many of us have denied ourselves the privilege and honor of feasting on His Word and His love. We are not coming to the table that He has so perfectly prepared for us. We have sought our own bread, the food of the world that offers temporary soothing, but never lasting peace. God made food for our enjoyment and nourishment, but He gave the life of His only Son to sustain us and empower us with spiritual food that would lead us to eternal life.

Deuteronomy 6:5 You shall love the LORD your God with all your heart, with all your soul, and with all your strength.

It's time to transfer our affections from food to God

There is unlimited peace in learning how to wait upon the Lord for our breakthrough and healing. When we worship, we give our full attention to God. He is glorified when we experience supernatural weight loss as our flesh shrinks in the presence of a Holy God. As we bask in God's glorious presence, our spirit man gets bigger and bigger as our flesh gets smaller and smaller. Our flesh is shrinking back and our spirit man is getting stronger. Worship is a tool for the believer who desires a closer fellowship with God and for people who desire breakthrough.

All promotion occurs in God's presence

When we witness changes and blessings come to pass in the natural, it is a direct reflection of how the heavens shifted during prayer and praise. Lasting joy lies in the recognition that God is more than adequate to fulfill our inner longings, and desires. Our abundance and our salvation were paid for on Calvary's Cross but there is truly victory in the praise! Our victory comes from being in the presence of the Lord. When we're in God's presence in a spirit of worship and praise, we experience breakthrough and freedom!

Psalm 145:3 Great *is* the LORD, and greatly to be praised; And His greatness *is* unsearchable.

When I put my focus on God and I make Him big, my problems get smaller. When I make God the center of my life and I focus on how large He is, how big His blessings are instead of how much weight I have to lose or how far I have to go, then I'm blessed.

Blessed because I realize that God is not limited to what I can see. I serve a mighty and awesome God. I can seek His abundance to fill me up so that I stop reaching for the counterfeit high of food and other addictions.

Isaiah 55:1-3 "Ho! Everyone who thirsts, Come to the waters; And you who have no money, Come, buy and eat. Yes, come, buy wine and milk Without money and without price. Why do you spend money for *what is* not bread, And your wages for *what* does not satisfy? Listen carefully to Me, and eat *what is* good, And let your soul delight itself in abundance. Incline your ear, and come to Me. Hear, and your soul shall live; And I will make an everlasting covenant with you— The sure mercies of David.

Why do we spend our money on what is not spiritual bread?

We run after the food of this world. We run after the pleasures of this world, we can be stuffed, but never satisfied. One of the greatest things that we could do is learn the difference between physical and spiritual hunger. So often when we feel hungry, we're really hungry for God's presence. We're confusing spiritual and physical hunger. The Psalmist says, as the deer panted for the water, so my soul longeth after thee (Psalm 42:1). Our hearts are crying out for fellowship. Yet, we are dragging our burdens to the *table* instead of to the *cross*. Worship is a part of spiritual warfare. We have been fighting the battle of obesity and the battle of overeating with the wrong weapons. We've been fighting with secular dieting and methods of this world, only to remain in a cycle of agony and disappointment.

2 Corinthians 10:4 For the weapons of our warfare *are* not carnal but mighty in God for pulling down strongholds

When I'm in God's presence, my transformation begins.

Praise is a mighty weapon that produces supernatural and natural changes. When I'm in God's presence, the Kingdom of Heaven opens up to answer my call for help. As believers, we are to be *heavy* in God's presence. In high worship, the weight of God's glory rests upon us. A moment in God's presence is worth more than a lifetime of self-effort. So, how long has it been that you've struggled with the bondage of overeating? How long has it been that you've tried everything that you can think of and yet nothing has worked?

A moment in God's presence can transform our entire lives

When we press into the presence of God, we have the attention of the Creator of the universe. In His presence, I find my elevation, provision, answer and weight loss solution. My works and actions, in the natural, only confirm what has already been accomplished through my worship.

Worship is communication with God

Genesis 3:8 And they heard the sound of the LORD God walking in the garden in the cool of the day, and Adam and his wife hid themselves from the presence of the LORD God among the trees of the garden.

Prayerlessness (hiding from God) began in the Garden of Eden.

Shame and guilt causes me to hide myself from God's presence. That's all the trick of the enemy because if he can keep me out of God's presence, then he can keep me away from my blessing and my breakthrough. The enemy can keep me from the healing and deliverance that comes from hearing and responding to God's voice.

Hebrews 4:15-16 For we do not have a High Priest who cannot sympathize with our weaknesses, but was in all *points* tempted as *we are, yet* without sin. Let us therefore come boldly to the throne of grace, that we may obtain mercy and find grace to help in time of need.

My spirit is hungry for reconciliation with God.

The phenomenal thing about Jesus is that there is nothing that I can struggle with, no thought, no temptation that Jesus has not already "been there, done that." By the time I get to Him in a position of prayer, He's basically saying, "Yep, I know." Jesus was without sin, but He is not without sympathy. He understands our struggles. He understands the battle. He also understands where our peace and success comes from and thus says, "Come boldly my daughter, come boldly my son into My presence, and you will get the grace and mercy to help you in your time of need." And when I empty out what's on the inside, I don't have to stuff it down with food. I don't have to stuff down the gnawing pain with food.

John 6:48 I am the bread of life.

My spirit is hungry for reconciliation with God. It's hungry for forgiveness, refreshing and intimacy with God. If I do not allow myself that time to be in His presence, then I will find other ways to feed that need. We run from God only to find ourselves tempted and led astray by destructive habits of the flesh. How has your spiritual food intake been? When we become *fat* in our spirits, we can choose to be lean in our physical appearance. God desires to fill us up with His spiritual food because our first need, remember, is always going to be for *living bread and water*. Our hunger is for more of Jesus.

Freedom from secret shame

A direct result of avoiding God's presence is shame. Shame is a key trigger for emotional eating and self-abuse. When we internalize shame, which is actually fear, we eat to numb the pain. And before you know it, we are just existing, not fully present nor passionately living to the fullness of each moment. There have been times in my life that I've been so checked out on food that I wake up three months later and wondered what I had been doing. And then my body and mind remind me that I've been eating! I've been eating and hiding from God. I hadn't been in connection and fellowship with Him. You show me a person who's consistently reaching for food to feed their flesh and I'll show you a person who is not connected with God on the level that God is calling them to be connected. There's a high calling of purpose and power on the lives of people who are in addictive cycles. God gave us an unquenchable thirst and insatiable hunger for Him. We have just gotten the hunger signal crossed. When we meet those needs for spiritual nourishment by consistently seeking God's wisdom and presence, we will rise to a level of confidence, beauty and passion that will even surpass our wildest dreams!

Are you having a private love affair with food?

I once heard a visiting youth pastor at our church say, "You go into a *private* place with your sin, because you have not been to the *secret* place with God." Many of us eat in private. We hide out and stuff our flesh. But God wants us to have a secret place where we communicate with Him; a place where we pray and give those hurts freely to His caring arms. When we refuse to bow down to the idol of food and instead worship the Living God, we will see the healing in our lives. We can seek God in that secret place and not have the temptation of going into a private place with our gluttony. When we first choose to feed our spirits in the secret place, the Lord becomes our divine source for nourishment.

Lose the inner weight and the outer weight will follow.

What is seen on the outside is just a reflection of the heaviness felt on the inside. In God's presence, clothed in a spirit of worship, we have the opportunity daily to lay our burdens down and cast our cares on a Savior who truly cares for us. There could be no better weight loss center than the throne room of the most High God. This is a place where we are guaranteed success, freedom and breakthrough. Through God's Word and the fellowship of worship, we find relief for our anxiety, comfort from disappointment and refreshing waters for the areas in our lives that have become dry and dead. In God's presence, we can feast on the bread of life that will sustain us for now and eternity. Worship is a most powerful weapon in the war against overeating and obesity. If I can become heavy with God's presence, then I can become light in weight. That's an awesome exchange!

Wellness through Worship

Matthew 9:20-22 And suddenly, a woman who had a flow of blood for twelve years came from behind and touched the hem of His garment. For she said to herself, "If only I may touch His garment, I shall be made well." But Jesus turned around, and when He saw her He said, "Be of good cheer, daughter; your faith has made you well."

And the woman was made well from that hour. For 12 years, this woman spent all of her resources. She went to every doctor that she could find. She went everywhere that she could and one touch from Jesus was worth more than 12 years of spending personal resources. Never undervalue the power of a moment in God's presence, for that is where we have God's full attention. This woman knew that if she could only touch Him, she would be made well. Jesus felt her faith and I believe He also felt her desperation for healing.

How desperate are you for God to heal you?

Are you desperate enough to set aside time to worship Him, to set aside time in the morning, afternoon or evening to come into His presence and praise Him? When I was in the battle to overcome overeating, I would lay before the Lord many a morning and night, crying out in desperation and pain, "Lord, please change me! Change my desire for the foods of this world. Give me a hunger for you only. Feed me Lord. Fill the void in my soul!" God revealed to me, while in His presence, that I was hungry for relief from rejection, hungry for acceptance, hungry for security and safety, hungry to feel His mighty touch and hungry for His love. I encourage you, as you seek to live by natural eating principles and overcome overeating and poor health, to make praise and worship an integral part of what you do. Our victory, weight loss and healing lie in God's presence.

CHAPTER TWELVE

Slim and Serene by Submission

I remember the first time I heard the word submission. The picture that came to my mind was a lowly weak woman, being abused by a strong burly man. That image was etched in my mind and I entered into Christianity somewhat fearful of submission and ignorant of the power of submission. From Joseph to Jesus, when you look in the Bible at all of the great men and women of faith, you see people who knew that in order to see God fully glorified, they needed to submit. They needed to stop fighting and defending themselves. One of the most beautiful women that I have the honor to have in my life is Sister Bunny Wilson. She's authored many powerful and popular books including *Liberated through Submission*. She also wrote that when we submit "God intervenes." I don't think there's anything more powerful that can be said about the principle of submission .When we submit to the plans and direction of God, we have the peace of God which passes all understanding. Submission is saying, "Lord, I trust your love, direction and plan for my life."

1 Peter 2:11-14 Beloved, I beg *you* as sojourners and pilgrims, abstain from fleshly lusts which war against the soul, having your conduct honorable among the Gentiles, that when they speak against you as evildoers, they may, by *your* good works which they observe, glorify God in the day of visitation. Therefore *submit yourselves* to every ordinance of man for the Lord's sake, whether to the king as supreme, or to governors, as to those who are sent by him for the punishment of evildoers and *for the* praise of those who do good (Italics mine).

God's Word says that we submit ourselves to authority. Charged with the responsibility of raising three boys, my husband and I are mindful of instilling in them a respect and submission to authority. When our sons submit to our authority, as parents, then they will understand submitting to the authority of teachers, leaders and ultimately to the authority of the Lord in their lives.

When we are submitted to God, then we are more willing to follow the commands of His Word, which also instruct us to be submitted to order and the natural laws here on earth (1Peter 2:13).

Jesus, the submitted man

Luke 22:42 saying, "Father, if it is Your will, take this cup away from Me; nevertheless not My will, but Yours, be done."

Jesus is our ultimate example of submission. He says, "Not My will, but Yours, be done." This is possibly the most painful time of His earthly life. This is before He faced the crucifixion and He knew everything that He was going to endure. He also knew for thousands and thousands of years to come that the very people that He would die on the cross for would be the ones who'd deny Him in their lives and lifestyle. He cried out earnestly to God. And even after He accepted God's will, the pain did not instantly cease. The Bible says that He wept more and more profusely until "his sweat became as drops of blood" (Luke 22:44). Jesus was, in His most human state, afraid of the pain that comes before the purpose of God is fulfilled. Yet, He reached a place of utmost submission and cried to the Father, "not My will, but Yours, be done." By accepting His own death, He gave life to every man who would ever call on His name.

Luke 22:45-46 When He rose up from prayer, and had come to His disciples, He found them sleeping from sorrow. Then He said to them, "Why do you sleep? Rise and pray, lest you enter into temptation."

Prayer empowers the principle of submission

If you're not in the place of constant prayer and communication with the Father, you will become tempted to go back and pick up that very thing that you've submitted and surrendered to the Lord. We lose the victory when we regress from submission into becoming managers and controllers of our lives. When we submit ourselves and our struggle with overeating to a Holy God, we take up our own cross and choose to *die daily* to the desires and dictates of our flesh. God moves us from bondage to wanting to preserve our comfort. He leads us to a place where we say daily, in our eating choices, "not my will but your will be done." Are you willing to submit daily to the plans God has for your life? Are you willing to lay down your dependency on the foods of this world and put your utmost trust in God for liberty and freedom? Submission to God's authority in our lives leads us to a place of elevation, new life and lasting victory.

The Spiritual Makeover

As believers, walking by God's Word for weight loss and wellness, we are experiencing a *spiritual extreme makeover* that will reveal itself in our natural body. Much like the caterpillar, we are inching towards our chrysalis, our place of utmost transformation. Before a caterpillar goes into the cocoon/chrysalis, he lives his life by two principles: *eating and survival*. Many of us have been fighting for so long to survive that we have forgotten how to live. We have, like the caterpillar, been in a cycle of eating and surviving, eating and surviving, yet God has called us into the transformation process. When we submit to purpose for our lives, the cocooning process begins. When the caterpillar enters the cocoon, it is dark, sticky, uncomfortable and unfamiliar, much like our healing process. Yet, on the other side is the butterfly. *The butterfly is the beautiful result of submission.*

It is good to survive, it is extraordinary to thrive!

Thriving in life is a by-product of submitting to the process of transformation and change. New creations in Christ, welcome the process of change, endure the unfamiliar and suffer the loss of comfort for the forming of our character, integrity and new life. When we emerge on the other side as beautiful butterflies, we will have a different view of life than we had as a caterpillar. We will see things from a higher view point. The caterpillar strives to survive and eats because he has a limited view. He only sees his immediate surrounding. To the contrary, the butterfly has vision. When we soar, by way of submission, our eyes are opened to see the purpose of God in our lives.

Submission is Patience

Even after we choose to submit to God, we must still endure the process of change. This requires patience. Most of us have a timeline requirement to meet our desires. We want everything right now! That's the society in which we live. We want it yesterday! Sometimes, we don't *feel* like God really hears us. We don't see God moving fast enough and in an attempt to manage pain and maintain some form of control over our environment, we control the food. Instead of submitting to God's perfect timing, we stuff the pain that comes from the inability to delay our gratification. We have forgotten what it is like to say *no* to ourselves. The pleasure of saying *yes* increases when it is balanced with the discipline of telling ourselves *no*.

Instant gratification increases long-term pain.

Psychologists say that Americans have lost touch with the healing art of tragedy and pain. In Shakespearean times, they were famous for their tragic plays because getting in touch with pain helped people to relish and welcome moments of sheer happiness. We live in a society that seeks pleasure, instant happiness and gratification. We live in a society that teaches us to avoid pain at all costs. How ironic that, in our society, depression, anxiety and stress-related hospitalization is at an alarming all time high. When we are impatient, we are deeply fearful that our most basic needs will not be met. When we overeat to provide instant gratification for our flesh, we are masking a deeper fear…our inability to trust God for His highest blessing.

Luke 21:19 By your patience possess your souls.

When we walk in patience, we can possess the circumstance and not let our circumstance possess us. As we learn to submit to God and wait upon the Lord, He will renew our strength (Isaiah 40:31). In the place of patience, we are in God's presence. And in God's presence, we are connected to His peace and His purpose. In God's presence, you're connected to the heart, purpose and mind of Christ. Patience says, "I already have what I need." The fear that drives impatience causes us to move outside of the Will of God. Because of impatience, we short-change ourselves by choosing to meet our own needs instead of waiting on God. Patience is not inactivity, just sitting around, waiting for God to do everything. Patience is a place of faith. Patience is a place of belief. Patience is a place where God is perfecting us.

James 1:2-4 My brethren, count it all joy when you fall into various trials, knowing that the testing of your faith produces patience. But let patience have *its* perfect work, that you may be perfect and complete, lacking nothing.

The diet world has fed into our pain and fear

The diet world promises quick, instant and effortless results, and as overeaters, we're impatient. We want the quick fix. We want the radical *Hollywood* overnight change. We want the quick fat loss diet plan. We are anxious for the *product* and sometimes fail to see God in the *process*. We want the pounds to fall off yesterday, but God's *inner weight loss plan* works on our character. He helps us break free from the fears and inconsistencies that have created the yo-yo weight gain and weight loss cycles. We want the quick fix, but God wants change in our hearts.

Lasting change comes from the process not the instant fix

If our hearts truly change during the process of healing, then we will keep the weight off permanently. Anyone can lose weight by manipulating food, but keeping it off is a different story. The facts are that 97-99% of diets fail to produce long term results. Trusting Jesus is not for people who want a quick fix. It is for people who truly want healing and the strength it takes to sustain their new bodies and lives. As you learn how to delay gratification, you will come to trust that *delay does not mean denial*. Later does not mean never. We serve a God whose Word does not return to Him void (Isaiah 55:11). When we submit to God's timing, we can trust that He is working things out. He is intervening on our behalf in ways that we cannot immediately see.

Isaiah 40:31 But those who wait on the LORD Shall renew *their* strength; they shall mount up with wings like eagles, they shall run and not be weary, they shall walk and not faint.

Submission is preparation

The book of Esther tells a powerful story of submission. It begins with a woman who refused to submit and thus lost her crown, her honor and all of the privileges of the kingdom. The book of Esther begins with a great feast that King Ahasuerus made for all of his princes and courtiers. The feast was to display the splendor and excellence on his kingdom. We pick up the story in verse 10.

Esther 1:10-12 On the seventh day, when the heart of the king was merry with wine, he commanded Mehuman, Biztha, Harbona, Bigtha, Abagtha, Zethar, and Carcas, seven eunuchs who served in the presence of King Ahasuerus, to bring Queen Vashti before the king, *wearing* her royal crown, in order to show her beauty to the people and the officials, for she *was* beautiful to behold. But Queen Vashti refused to come at the king's command *brought* by *his* eunuchs; therefore the king was furious, and his anger burned within him.

Vashti did not submit to the King. She did not submit to the possibilities of the kingdom. He was one of the richest, most powerful rulers on earth. To have his favor would have given Vashti access to anything her heart desired, but she failed to submit to a simple request that had monumental consequences. The King is symbolic of God in our own lives. He wants to show our beauty, our light, our gifts to the world and we tell him *no* by our behavior. When we are not fully submitted to God's plan for our lives, we can compromise our position of honor and purpose, much like Vashti did. The story continues to explain that Vashti was banned from the kingdom and lost her rights to her land and authority. She lost access to the beauty and the blessings of this rich kingdom. The king, instructed by the counsel of his trusted advisors, set out to find a Queen that was "better than Vashti."

Esther, a gentle and submitted beauty

We are then introduced to Esther, a woman wise and powerful enough to submit to God's plan for her destiny as well as the people that God placed in positions of authority that would help propel her to her rightful place of honor and influence. Esther, whose original name was Hadassah, was raised by Mordecai. She was his uncle's daughter and the Bible says that she had neither father nor mother. The Bible speaks of Esther's overwhelming beauty, but it also speaks of her untouchable spirit of meekness and humility. Esther's life was not only purposed for greatness, it was shaped by favor.

Esther 2:8 And so it was, when the king's command and decree were heard, and when many young women were gathered at Shushan the citadel, under the custody of Hegai, that Esther also was taken to the king's palace, into the care of Hegai the custodian of the women.

Esther's submission to God invited unlimited favor

I wondered how many of those women murmured and complained about being taken into the custody of Hegai. Did they all go willingly? Did some fight? Did some not want to leave the comfort and connection to family? Esther had lost her father and mother years ago and the Bible did not speak of her having any brothers or sisters, so I believe she humbly accepted the invitation. She was not tied to the cares of the world like many of the other women could have been. I believe Esther's spirit was different. There was something that set her apart. The favor of God was present in her life as she consistently submitted, knowing that God was using those in authority to bless and promote her.

Esther 2:9 Now the young woman pleased him, and she obtained his favor; so he readily gave beauty preparations to her, besides her allowance. Then seven choice maidservants were provided for her from the king's palace, and he moved her and her maidservants to the best *place* in the house of the women.

Submission changes your environment

Esther's willingness to submit to God's best for her life paid off, in dividends of favor, with those charged to care for her. She was given additional treatments and moved to an environment that would not place her in the immediate surroundings of jealously, competition and contempt that the other women may have felt for her. When we submit to God's plan for our lives, the favor and elevation that follows may cause us to separate from people, situations and environments that do not propel us towards destiny. We must pray on our journey towards wholeness and healing that we are surrounded by people who are partnering with us in purpose, and helping us to see the plan of God come to pass in our lives.

Esther 2:12 Each young woman's turn came to go in to King Ahasuerus after she had completed twelve months' preparation, according to the regulations for the women, for thus were the days of their preparation apportioned: six months with oil of myrrh, and six months with perfumes and preparations for beautifying women.

How much time will you invest in submission to God's plan?

Most of us find it hard to give up a few hours on Sunday for worship at our churches. We also find it difficult to give up the time to exercise, the time it takes to read labels, cook food at home or give our bodies rest and relaxation. In the body of Christ, we sometimes focus too much on the spiritual and do not realize that God is a God who uses natural circumstances to advance His purpose. In this case, He not only used Esther's gentle spirit, but also the incredible beauty that she was blessed with at birth. Beauty that went to an entirely different level once her 12 months of purification and beauty treatments were complete.

The world spends time and money on what is perishing

In Hollywood, actresses spend thousands and thousands of dollars and countless hours on a weekly basis to beautify themselves and showcase their beauty to a fallen world. And yet, when God calls us to prepare ourselves for His purpose and greatness to be revealed, we resist. Women in the world put more care and attention into a body that does not even house the Holy Spirit of God and we neglect and abuse His temple, a place that is to be fully submitted to God. Are you willing to allow God to beautify you inside and out? Are you willing to let go of destructive habits in your flesh that compromise your physical beauty and health? Esther submitted to the process of beautification and we must also surrender, in obedience, to the process of transformation from the inside out. We must do this so that the unlimited favor and beauty of God will manifest in our lives.

Esther is elevated because of submission

Esther 2:13-17 Thus *prepared, each* young woman went to the king, and she was given whatever she desired to take with her from the women's quarters to the king's palace. In the evening she went, and in the morning she returned to the second house of the women, to the custody of Shaashgaz, the king's eunuch who kept the concubines.

She would not go in to the king again unless the king delighted in her and called for her by name. Now when the turn came for Esther the daughter of Abihail the uncle of Mordecai, who had taken her as his daughter, to go in to the king, she requested nothing but what Hegai the king's eunuch, the custodian of the women, advised. And Esther obtained favor in the sight of all who saw her. So Esther was taken to King Ahasuerus, into his royal palace, in the tenth month, which *is* the month of Tebeth, in the seventh year of his reign. The king loved Esther more than all the *other* women, and she obtained grace and favor in his sight more than all the virgins; so he set the royal crown upon her head and made her queen instead of Vashti.

Esther's entire life and destiny was transformed in one instant

We have the ability to prepare for the moments in our lives when God will use our preparation to meet with His opportunity. This is where we will find favor and success. When we, like Esther, submit and say, "Lord, not my will, but Your will be done." Your will be done for my family. Your will be done for my life. Your will be done for my health and my eating habits. We will then see the elevation and promotion in our lives as we also see the transformation of our bodies.

Submission is humility

James 4:6-7 But He gives more grace. Therefore He says: *"God resists the proud, But gives grace to the humble."* Therefore submit to God. Resist the devil and he will flee from you.

You show me a humble person and I'll show you a submitted person. Humble simply means "being oneself" when I no longer have an image to protect or uphold my life is truly submitted and the real authentic woman shines through. If people tell me I am humble when they meet me, they are simply saying to me that I am being myself. There was a time that I was "not myself." I was living life based on what my selfish ambition dictated I *should* be. I was miserable and proud. I know firsthand that God resists me when I'm proud. He doesn't hear me when I'm proud. His hand is against me when I'm proud, but He gives me more grace when I'm humble. I see more of the manifestation of His glory, His provision and His blessing in my life when I live a submitted life.

Obedience to God's will and natural laws is worship

Perhaps, you wonder what to do now at the closing of this book. I would encourage you to submit. Submit to the wisdom of the teachings that have been laid out before you. Submit daily to the natural laws of hunger and fullness that God put in place to regulate, tone your body and strengthen your health. *Listed below*:

One: Waiting on and responding to True Physical Hunger. Eating only when you are truly physically hungry. Not from mental hunger, not from emotional hunger, not from spiritual hunger, but from true physical (stomach) hunger.

Two: Eating to the point of comfortable satisfaction. We will not gorge or stuff ourselves to the point of pain, discomfort, self-abuse or gluttony.

Three: Wise Eating. Using and exercising wisdom in my personal eating choices. Taking responsibility over my own health and food choices and eating the foods that are agreeable and favorable to my body.

And finally, submit to whatever the Lord is instructing you to do in a very personal sense through His Word or in your time of quiet fellowship. Obedience is above all sacrifice (1Samuel 15:22). It is also one of the highest forms of worship. So, when I say, "Lord, I'm submitting to Your will for my marriage, my career path, my purpose and my finances. I'm submitting to Your will when it comes to the way I treat my body temple." I will see the blessing of God as well as the favor and peace of God in my life.

We gain a better body by obedience.

I will see the manifestation of a new body because I'm not living according to *my* will that has led me down a path of discouragement and disappointment. I am living according to God's Word, fully submitted to Him and knowing that when I'm submitted, God intervenes on my behalf.

A final note:

On your journey, please be patient, gentle and loving to yourself. Success is not overnight. You will fall, but God will lift you back up. You may stumble, but God will restore you to a place of faith and hope. This is not a diet. There is no black and white or extreme thinking of good and bad. I only encourage you to not give up on the dreams you have for total restoration and new life. We serve a God who cares so deeply for us. I believe that along the way of discovering yourself, you will discover even more greatly the depths of His love. Remember, God is not concerned with the size of our bodies, but the size of our hearts. Will you give Him your heart completely? Will you allow Him access to the secret and hidden places of pain? Will you allow the transforming work of Calvary's Cross to resurrect the dead places in your soul? It's time for new life. It's time for freedom. It's time to declare to a dying world that:

Diets don't work...But Jesus does.

Printed in the United States
109599LV00003B/253/A